God Bless Modern Medicine

ISBN: 978-93-88660-73-0

Published and Printed by:
Sankalp Publication
Head Office: Ring Road 2 Gaurav Path, Bilaspur,
Chhattisgarh – 495001
Phones: +91 9111395888 +91 9111396888
Email: support@sankalppublication.com
Website: www.sankalppublication.com

God Bless Modern Medicine.

Vaid Atwal

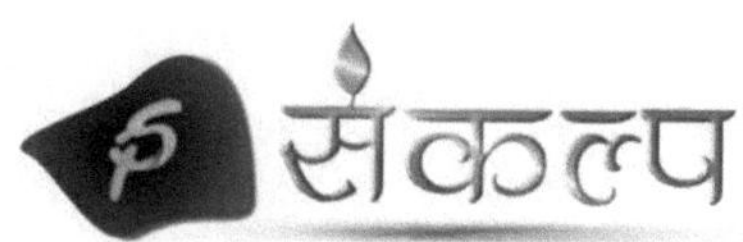

Vaid Atwal's
God Bless Modern Medicine

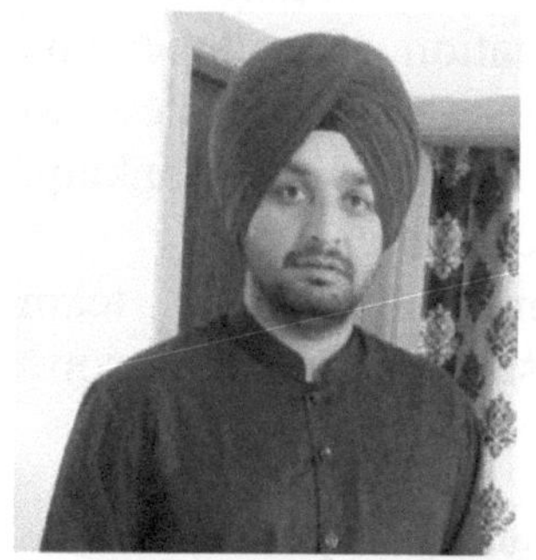

Author- Vaid Atwal
(Ayurvedic Physician)

Writing assisted by:

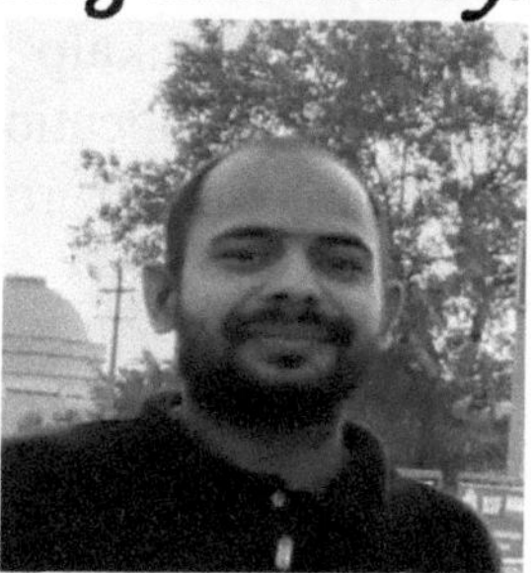

Dr. Sandeep Kumar

Sankalp Publication team

Publishing is a media to express the think of person between society and author. Our Publishing team are providing many information. we hope this information will benefit those who are new to publishing. Publishing process with Sankalp, simplified your publishing requirement.

On Sankalp Publication Have Many team members, we inform you mostaly dedicated person.

Sheela Yadav - Sales Department
Aakash Rahore - Publishing Department
Jainarayan Kaiwart - Digital Department
Chitrakant Sao - Distribution Department
Rajesh Banjare - Order Department

Sankalp team member are inpired by author feedback. Sankalp are supporting liftime there author for Publication Services. Our Publication are given maximum royalty compare to other book publication.

Dedication

This book is dedicated to my parents firstly without whom; I might not be at the position where I am today. After them, I would like to dedicate this book to the person who himself dedicated his whole life in serving humanity. I am lucky enough for having the prestigious opportunity to learn under such a legendary physician & the Master healer who changed and influenced my life in many ways. I bow my head before, *"Late Vaidya P.Y. Vaidya Khadiwale"*. His significant efforts have benefitted the society in many ways.

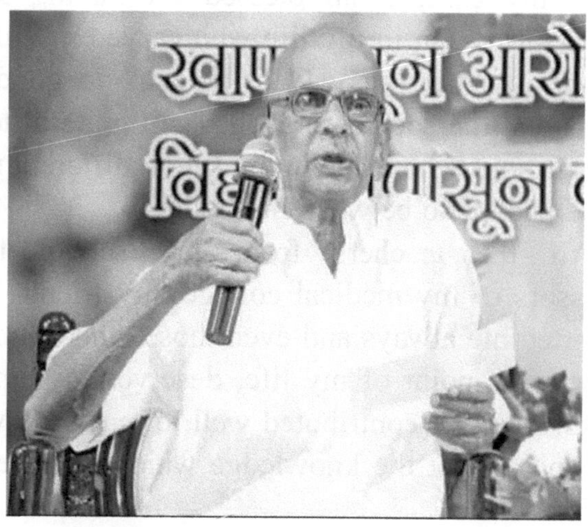

Late Vaidya P.Y. Vaidya Khadiwale.
250-D, Shaniwar Peth,
Pune, Maharashtra.

Acknowledgement

When a child is born, he/she is like an empty book or a blank diary. In difficult stages of life, this diary starts reflecting the impression of various persons who knowingly or unknowingly designs some pages or chapters of that book. With time, different persons pay their contribution in completing this book, what we call life. Good writers write some fantastic pages in the book of your life whereas, if those people are toxic in any sense, this life book could be horrible.

In my case, I am blessed for having some wonderful person in my life who carved my life in such a way that today I am able to do good for myself and the society as well. I am grateful to all those persons who came in my life in different roles and helped me to be what I am today.

All the teachers from my school time, professors of my medical college, my friends who supported me always and even those who criticized me at some point of my life, deserves my sincere thanks. They all contributed well to make me work hard and collect the knowledge which is presented in this book.

Vaid Ranpreet Singh Atwal
Ayurvedic Expert, Physician & Author

Foreword

It is really a mixed feeling of privilege and pleasure to write few words as foreword on the book "God Bless Modern Medicine" by 'Vaid Ranpreet Singh Atwal'. With this book, author has achieved another milestone. Vaid Atwal has also written a famous book "Naadi Abhayas" based on ancient Ayurvedic Science of pulse diagnosis in year 2015. With overwhelming success of his first mission as a writer, he has again penned a new book for his readers discussing fundamentals of Modern medicine which are crucial for healthy life of mankind. Although, we all are aware of contributions made by Modern medicine to the society and we also appreciate that. As we all know, modern science is continuously developing with time but certain fundamental principles are time tested. Author as a reader of modern science found some interesting facts about this science related to healthcare which are undermined by practitioners these days. As someone once said that, "Health science has advanced so much that nobody is healthy now". Healthy life is a result of healthy diet and lifestyle. So, present book is author's expression of thoughts as a scholar.

Vaid Atwal is very close friend of mine. He is charismatic personality with multiple talents. Although as a busy physician, he still manages to find time for reading and writing books, blogs and health related articles, delivers guest lecture to promote health status of the society by educating the masses and he also trains aspiring doctors with all the good deeds as a mentor. 'Vaid Atwal' has a hunger for knowledge and he works very hard to satisfy his quest. His effort reminds me a famous verse of 'Charak Samihita':

sastram jyotih prakasartham darsanam buddhiratmanah/ tabhyam bhisak suyuktabhyam cikitsannaparadhyati//
Cikitsite trayah pada yasmadvaidyavyapasrayah/ tasmat prayatnamatisthedbhisak sragunasampadi//

Which means, "Scientific scriptures provide light for illumination (to remove darkness of ignorance or to know things) and once own intellect is like eyes. The physician who use both (Scientific knowledge and own intellect) properly and doesn't commit mistakes during treatment. Hence physician should make all efforts to enrich his qualities.

I wish him great success with this book and for future aims as well.

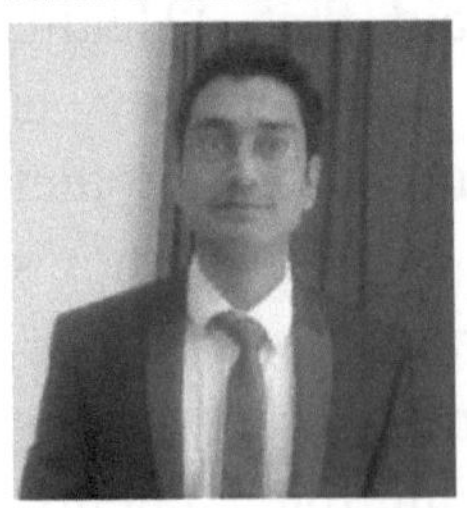

Dr. Keshav Rana
Ex. Asitt. Professor
(Babe ke Ayurvedic College,
Moga, Punjab)
Currently serving as:
Medical Officer
(Himachal Pradesh Govt.)

Some opinions about Author & Expectations from This Book

1.

This book is going to be a perfect milestone for all the medical professionals like us; Medical students and public in general. He is a great mentor and a coach as he works on the rudimentary concepts of medical practice & health science. We must be thankful to Vaid Atwal for presenting such a valuable book. His words reflect his deep understanding and experience regarding this field. He is a great influencer and an inspirational personality for all the persons interested in wellbeing of human body and all those who are concerned with medical field

Dr. Tapasya Sharma
(Ayurvedic Physician & Panchkarm Consultant)
Dr. Abhishek Sharma
(Ayurvedic Surgeon & Ano-rectal disease specialist,
Founder & Owner MRC Ayurveda, Vrindaban, U.P India)

2.

Vaid Ranpreet Singh Atwal is dynamic personality and he is working tirelessly. This is second book by author, after the huge success of his first book. In this book, he has presented the modern medicine in an honest way without the aim of criticizing modern medicine. His main intention is to draw the attention of more and more people towards actual and authentic way of healing.

I wish him all the success for new endeavors.

Dr. Prashant Sood
[B.A.M.S, M.S-Ayu. (ENT Dept.)]
Professor: SKSS Ayurvedic College,
Sarabha, Ludhiana (Pb.)

3.

As they say, "**Curiosity is the mother of all inventions and advancements**". The modern medical science is a result of curiosity of mankind for a faster way of treatment of rather management of diseases. But to match this fast paced life, we are creating more disasters on the name of treatments. This book uncovers a lot of myths and secrets about the modern medicine which has grown from being an alternate form of medicine to a main stream line pathy, suppressing all the natural form of treatments. The author has made a firm attempt to enlighten the readers to think and act on facts that are seldom known rather than own myths.

I wish him all the best for this book and all his future endeavors.

Dr. Unique Sharma
[Final year P.G. Scholar
Department of Panchkarma
SDM College of Ayurveda & Hospital
Hassan, Karnataka (India)]

4.

It is quite difficult to write down the qualities of such a mentor in words. However, Vaid Ranpreet Singh Atwal is the one whom I met a decade ago as a regular batch mate. He is a man with stupendous cognizance and special abilities to apprehend a complex concept in a simple perceivable way so that, it seems interesting and easy to the others. He loves to render his ideology and point of view regarding any concept to his students, so that, they can also use his methods while treating patients.

"WORDS SPEAK LOUDER THAN VOICE". So he confined his thoughts in his book, "GOD BLESS MODERN MEDICINE" where he has revealed the truth of rampant anecdotal myths about health. It will surely mesmerize the person who is curious about health and health sciences. Being an Ayurvedic physician, he confers logical scientific research (not modern medicine) for a long healthy life with a fusion of both ancient and modern science.

It is a miniscule statement that I can give about him.

Dr. Amanpreet Singh
(Ayurvedic Physician)
Owner-Ojas health care Centre
Dohara, (Ludhiana) Punjab.

Disclaimer

- ✓ This book is not against any particular organisation, association or any individual.
- ✓ This book is only to recall basic fundamental science required for a healthy living and this is not a medical textbook either.
- ✓ This book is only meant for putting a light on unfair health dogma which is ruining health of our society and spreading misinformation only for business. This is not only damaging health but also plundering money at the same time.
- ✓ I believe body is self-healing, self-repairing machine created by God. Medicine can only help to speed up the recovery process of body. But medicating lifelong just to fix some symptoms only by completely ignoring the science behind these abnormalities is definitely unfair.
- ✓ Neither this book is supposed to defame any particular pathy nor its motive is to unfairly favour any pathy, this book is only meant to benefit the society by awareness about the science of healing.
- ✓ Author is not funded by any organisation, pathy or institution to spread any agenda.

Vaid [signature]

About Author

Vaid Atwal has started his journey of being a doctor from his very early days. When the other students were choosing their subjects under the guidance of their parents, he himself selected the medical field with the dream of becoming a doctor. He always has a different approach regarding disease from his teenage and his passion towards his work is really unmatchable.

During the college time, he was not in that standard race of cramming books, just to get good grades. In fact, he has started studying various books regarding medical profession from different sources. His knowledge never confined up to syllabus and traditional learning styles in medical colleges. When he started practicing after the completion of his studies, he started treating patients with his different approach resulting, he was treating very difficult and some untreatable cases with very basic concepts of health. He is so curious in collecting and spreading knowledge that during the time of his higher studies in Pune, he has a thought to write a book and spread the knowledge that he has gained. So, in the very early age he had written his first book on a very tough and significant topic of pulse diagnosis.

Being an Ayurvedic physician, he reads modern science, latest researches and collaborate it with ancient science to give a logical reason for every query of his patient. So, in this book he has shared some unseen and ignored points of modern science with the logical example: Truth about cholesterol; Role of blood pH in disease; Sick effects of antibiotics and many more. Readers will definitely see a different point of view while reading this book. He has tried to explain it in a very simple way so everyone, who is not even from medical background, can easily understand it. He has given an ample data about many concepts.

He loves to travel different areas and explore the living and eating habits of that particular area and gather knowledge. He prevail diet over medicine and tries to educate his patients also. His preference in treatment is to get rid the patients from medicine and give them a perfect life without medications for lifetime. His different approach and practice style can also be seen in his social media platforms, he handles where he started educating and revealing the hidden truths of medical field.

Special thanks to Dr. Amanpreet Singh for writing such a descriptive "About Author" section of this book.

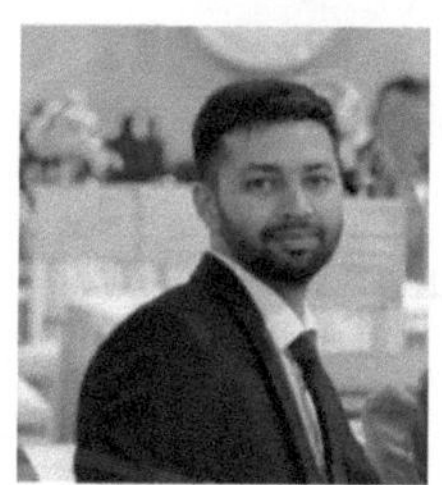

Dr. Amanpreet Singh
(Ayurvedic Physician)
Owner: OJAS HEALTH CARE CENTRE.
Doraha (Ludhiana) Punjab

Content

Introduction

God Bless Modern Medicine

This book is a result of my curiosity towards medical profession. This book will give you a new idea about health, disease and our conventional approach to manage any disease. The traditional way of looking at any disease is very limited and narrow. I must say, with all the advancements in medical profession we are still sick as a society.

We have advanced machines, gadgets, hi-tech laboratories, other diagnostic ways and all those stuff which we were having never before but is it worth? Can we say that we had given our society a wonderful health?

Honestly, if someone asks me have we developed advanced machines for medical aid, my answer will be YES. Have we moved ahead in research section of disease and health, my answer will be a YES AGAIN. Have we developed advanced surgical techniques & medicine, it's again a YES. But are we healthier & able to eradicate diseases permanently. Griefly, I have to admit that it is not working.

So genuinely, a question arises in our minds that where we went wrong? Are there any points which is important and we are still not working on that. Yes, we have forgotten basic science & physiology that how this body works. This book is my effort to recall all those basic principles, science

& biochemistry, so that our approach towards any diseases could be transformed in a fruitful way.

Just look at the graph of diseases in our society and our advancements in last 100 years, your head will definitely ring.

The pattern which is coming ahead is destroying our so called advancement in medical profession. On the one hand, we are blowing a trumpet of our success in developing latest advanced machines, robotic surgical arms & advanced medical procedure. Contrastingly, on the other hand, our health concerns is moving from minor issues to a lifelong condition for which we have to take number of drugs daily just to keep it balanced.

So, this book is a journey from not knowing to knowingness, ignorant to education & ultimately from unhealthiness to a completely healthy state of body & mind.

Chapter – I
Blood - River of Life

As we all know, blood is the vital fluid of our body & it delivers number of functions. Some of these functions are so common that it needs not to be discussed here because I expect that if you are reading this book we need not to talk about, rudimentary & very commonly known functions of the blood. Which includes transfers of nutrition from one portion to another, absorption of nutrition from our food, transfer of vital gases during respiration & many more. What I will be talking here is not very common & majority of medical professionals may not be aware of this. But these ignored functions are creating mess out of our lives. So let's discuss this in details.

Our body carries around 4-5 liters of blood and it has a pH of 7.2 to 7.4. This pH is very important because it is so vital if by any reason, your pH drops by only one unit i.e. up to 6 or increases by one unit from its normal expected value. Let's assume it become 8. In both the cases, you will be either in coma or dead.

Which means, you are living only if your blood is maintaining its pH very keenly. Only up & down just by one unit can screw you up completely. But don't worry here is a good news. Your body can never allow this to happen. By any method, you can't change your pH of blood. In fact, if you intentionally try this, by taking 100 percent acidic food or 100 percent basic food, your body's buffer system will come in action & it will keep your blood pH within range. So how is this happening, this is a very important question here.

Buffer System:

Body has certain departments which work accordingly to keep your blood pH within range. First is respiratory system.

As your body detects high acid in blood which is also called acidosis. Your body will immediately detect it & command your respiratory system to increase respiration rate. So that, more & more oxygen can be brought into your blood & heavy amount of CO2 could be expelled out. Oxygen is basic in nature, which means it cuts acid from the blood whereas, CO2 is acidic in nature it contributes in acidosis & keeps acid levels high in blood. So, when your body increases respiration rate, body is trying to cut excess acid from blood by intake of extra amount of oxygen & throwing out extra amount of CO2 from the blood. This acidosis condition could be seen in many diseases which indicate that your disease is associated with higher acid levels in blood.

Second system, which acts under buffer system, is your excretory organ that is your kidneys. Kidneys are the organs which filters your blood continuously, approximately in every 24 hours 7000-8000 liters of blood passes through kidneys for filtration. Out of which 1.5 to 2 liter of excess salts, minerals & water are thrown out of the body in the form of urine. If your blood is too acidic your kidney will start throwing acid contents out of your body in urine which will contribute to bring those acid levels down.

Third system, which helps to keep blood pH normal, is our skin. Skin is the largest organ in our body, which is very important to keep the blood pH in optimum range. Skin not only looks at pH of blood but it also regulates temperature of our body. Your skin also throws some water, some gases & very little amount of salts out of your body. This also maintains our constant internal temperature & helps blood to be in its normal state.

Fourth system, which works under your buffer system, is your G.I.T (Gastro Intestinal Tract) when you eat any meal it gets digested in stomach & small intestine. Whatever you eat has direct impact on your blood. In fact, everything your body carries is absorbed from the food you have eaten. This system is also influenced by disturbed blood pH. In alkaline state or in basic state of blood, your body will tend to pick acidic substance from G.I.T. & vice-versa. It means if your blood pH is running out of its harmony your G.I.T. will contribute to have that balance back by selecting what to absorb & what not. If your blood goes acidic your body will not absorb the nutrients which will contribute to acid and shows acidic effect in blood. This is the whole idea of pH & how body keeps it balanced.

Buffer Emergency:

It is a state when your body cannot balance its pH of blood by previously mentioned routine buffer actions. Then body declares an emergency state, which I believe is buffer emergency state. I call it buffer emergency because during this state your body behaves exactly the way when it's a national emergency in a country. No rules will be followed, all regular metabolic paths will be altered, loss to body will not be calculated and the only motive of the body will be to bring the pH of blood back in range. This is happening because body has a survival threat now. Body cannot bear or withstand the fluctuations in pH of blood. Let's assume you are in a state where your pH of blood tends to shift towards acidic, what your body will need now is basic substances to neutralize excess acid. One of the strongest base in your body is Calcium. Your body will firstly try to absorb maximum amount of Calcium from G.I.T. into blood but if your body fails to do so for any reason e.g. you might not be having required amount of Calcium in diet & the body is failing to neutralize it through lungs & kidneys. Then it's really an emergency condition for body. Now, body will behave in a different manner to keep things normal & survive. Your body is now ready to pay a price for this Calcium deficiency. Your body will now snatch Calcium from your bones & bring it back to blood because Calcium is the strongest base element that your body has. Body will not care about your bone health now. Your body is designed to survive at any cost, if you will not give it Calcium from your diet, body will forcefully snatch it from your bones.

Now let's assume, you are still ignorant or your physician cannot objectify the fault with your blood pH & you don't change your life style & eating habits, what will happen next will be even more dangerous. Your body will keep extracting Calcium from bones continuously which will trouble you in many ways. Firstly, less Calcium in bones may cause joint problems like osteoporosis or many other related problems. On the other hand, excess Calcium in the body which is floating freely in your blood is another threat for you. It can cause a troubled condition to you in number of ways. If this extra Calcium of blood got stuck in your kidneys, it will cause stones in your kidneys or if it gets into your heart and binds there or sediment in your arteries the consequences could be fatal as it could even cause infract or heart attack. If you are throwing chemicals in your blood stream by modern medicine, this whole process will proceed faster as most of modern medicine are basically chemical based and will eventually increase acid in your blood.

Nowadays, this acidic condition of blood is very common because we are being bombarded with acid causing foods from every side. Many doctors rely or depend on blood calcium levels for checking bones health or normal Calcium level for various health conditions. But now you know well, if your body is under buffer emergency; you will get very wrong information. Being Calcium deficient, your blood Calcium levels will be normal or slightly raised. If your doctor is ignorant, he might advise you not to focus on Calcium in your diet but this is very wrong approach. Some types of skin allergies are also caused when your acid level in blood is raised & instead of looking at the cause you go for anti-allergic or steroidal medication for regular basis. What you are doing here is totally against your body. These anti allergic medicines will increase more acid in your blood though your skin allergy is suppressed but you are in a big trouble now, within few months or years you can face a bigger health issue related to blood pH.

For your more understanding, I would like to discuss one of my patients here. A lady of approximately 35 years visited my office with complaints of hair fall, premature grey hairs, renal calculus and many more. She used to take some medicines for this & calculus is gone but within few months renal stones reappear. She is also having chronic UTI, skin rashes, burning micturition, headache, general fatigue, loud respiration, grade-2 fatty liver, elevated blood pressure & increased heart rate. She was getting treatment from reputed hospital in her vicinity & what doctors had prescribed her surprised me. She was prescribed hair oil, some medicines for renal calculus, anti-biotic for UTI, anti-allergic medicines for skin rashes, some syrups for burning micturition, some painkillers for headache, some multivitamins & respiratory pump. Not only this, she was also on an anti-hypertensive drug to be taken daily for blood pressure & I was speechless. That doctor was totally clueless as he was simply throwing a medicine for each symptom. All the symptoms could be tied to single cause and that is increased acid level in blood. I checked her serum Calcium report that was raised high. I explained that patient about her condition that you are carrying higher acid levels in your blood. An increased Calcium level in blood is also indicating that your body has stolen this Calcium from your bones, which is not only harmful for your bones but for rest of the vital organs as well. I dragged her attention from symptoms to root cause & convinced her to change her dietary habits from acidic to alkaline. Some herbal medicines were prescribed for one week & called her back after a week to report. She was drastically improved and after two months of proper medication and diet modification she was totally recovered. All her medications were discontinued afterwards and advised to keep an eye on her diet in future. This patient was struggling from last 3-4 years with these symptoms and was getting trapped deeper day by day. She was also surprised that she was misdiagnosed earlier & this is happening to a very big section of our society.

Practical aspect of blood pH:

Though it seems like a simple concept when we are discussing about blood pH. If the blood pH is going towards acidic, we know we need base in our diet or alkaline foods & things will be fixed. But it is not that simple, the problem with our modern science is we rely more than anything on our modern diagnostic methods say pH of blood (Lab. Test). There are many diseases which develop in our body due to higher acid tendencies, but we have no method to detect it from blood test. This is the point which confuses us because your body is working continuously to keep your blood pH in normal range as discussed previously. Our modern doctors are trained either to suppress a symptom or to balance blood reports & in this process the cause of the disease remains unnoticed & untouched. There are many diseases which are caused by acid environment in the body but we are increasing that acid even more with allopathic medicines and the cause of those diseases is not addressed. Change in blood pH is only visible in blood reports when the buffer system of your body surrenders & your body is not designed to surrender till its last breath. Let's dive into an example to have more understanding about what I am trying to explain here.

Fungal infection or Leucorrhoea (white discharge in women):

pH of female vagina is 3.8 -4.5 and pH of uterus is 6.5-7.6. Any kind of bacterial or fungal growth will grow here only if by any cause female body fails to keep this pH within required range. Even if vagina is exposed to any fungal infection this pH will kill those pathogens and infection can't grow. On the other hand, if a female is having more acidic food in diet (soft drinks, hard drinks, bread, pasta, various kind of sauce, packed, junk food, preserved food, fried and spicy food) she is very prone to develop these infection. But being a pH related problem doctors can't detect or identify this as a blood pH problem because this will not be visible in your blood reports as evidence. Instead of advising the patient to avoid acid causing food and switch to alkaline fresh and plant based diet, the doctor will prescribe some anti-fungal drugs. So, what is happening here? Let's understand. Antifungal drugs may kill the fungal infection for a short period but being a chemical base medicine this will contribute to increase more acid in body which results in recurrent fungal infections again and again because doctor missed to address the root cause and ignorantly he is contributing to feed the cause.

I had seen many patients visited my office with these fungal infections. Most of them have same statement that when we take antifungal medicines, symptoms disappear temporarily but it strikes back again and again. Most of them are struggling from years with same problem. I wonder how ignorance of modern doctors is creating a mess for a simple and easily treatable condition. This is an example almost in every disease such mistakes are being repeated by our trained doctors of modern medical system.

Kidney Failure, Albuminuria & Blood PH Link:
As per national kidney foundation 10 percent of the population worldwide is affected by chronic kidney disease (CKD) & millions of patients die every year because they do not have access to affordable treatments. In 1990, according to global Burdon of diseases study, Chronic Kidney Disease was ranked at 27th place in the list of worldwide death and in 2010 it rose to 18th in the same list which means in 20 years kidney disorders have speeded up & affected a bigger section of our world. Till 2010, there were mainly 5 countries having maximum number of CKD but in last 10 years India is now 6th country in this list. Now it is estimated that more than 850 million people worldwide are having kidney diseases which is a big number to declare kidney disorders as epidemic.

This also means that all the modern medicines and procedures we are having for kidney problems are actually useless. Governments of all countries are investing huge amount of money every year in this direction but unfortunately, we are still not having a reliable line of treatment to improve kidney functions. The reason is our approach & understanding towards kidney disease is totally wrong. Kidney performs mainly two functions, first one is filtration of blood which is known to everyone & second one is regulating blood pH which is majorly ignored by our modern medical system.

As far as kidneys are concerned, it is designed to work for you throughout your lifetime. It will only alter its way of working, if we put our system out of its pH zone. It is often seen that when kidneys shows primary symptoms of its damage we fail to understand its cause. Not only is this, the medicines our modern medical system offers us is totally against the system of our body. Let's discuss some disordered conditions to understand this concept with a wider angle.

Albuminuria:

It is a condition when your kidneys are throwing out amino acids or albumins out from your body. In this condition, laboratory investigations show the presence of albumin in urine. Now I want you to emphasis on the way, how I described albuminuria. I said that your kidneys are throwing out amino acids or albumins out of the body and modern science will define it as a condition when your nephrons (glomerulus) opening becomes dilated and these bigger molecules of albumins passes through them into urine. Both statements represent or admit presence of albumins in urine but for different reasons. The way how modern medical system describes this condition reveals their understanding. They are defining it in a wrong way. Ask any doctor, if he could explain why these glomerulus openings are dilated, they can't explain this. Now let's look on this condition in a scientific way which could make sense. If someone is having more acid in his blood which could not be balanced by routine buffer action of blood, your body will see this excess acid in blood as a life threat now. In order to survive your body has to throw out essential amino acids from the body because as the name indicates amino acids are basically acidic molecules which are carried in blood and making blood acidic. For survival reasons, your body will unwillingly throws them out to get its normal pH value back & work properly. You will be amazed to know most of the patients having albuminuria are diagnosed further as a chronic renal failure condition. What if I say, having alkaline food, Oxygen rich fresh air & deep breath, some required herbal medicines for providing base to the blood can heal this condition within weeks. Can you agree with this? Does it make sense to you that diseases caused by acidic environment could be treated with basic herbs and food items? Is it really that simple for which our huge medical system of healthcare is failing so badly and bigger section of country's economy is being drained out only to treat such renal disorders. If yes, then you are absolutely right. Now let me explain what allopathic doctors are doing for this, they are just trying to reduce pressure towards kidney by dilating blood vessels with a chemical tablet named "Ramipril". They really missed the science and physiology of the body here. Throwing out amino acids was an intelligent response of your body towards increased acid levels in blood. But treating acids with again some kind of allopathic medicines will make the diseases even more worse. Along with all the side effects this tablet (ramipril) will offer you; you are also hurting your kidneys even more and within few years, this condition may convert into serious health disorder like chronic renal failure (CRF). Some practitioners behave even more foolish and also attach some kind of antibiotic within their prescriptions. God knows who told them that bacteria are responsible for all this and antibiotics will help in such condition. My sincere sympathy towards all the patients of such extraordinary doctors!

What are the real threats of having an Acidic Body:

Having acid in blood or excess acid at cellular level can damage various systems of our body by many ways. Most of the biochemical reactions necessary for proper functioning of body got hampered in acidic medium. Our blood is slightly basic and it wants to be like that. Most of the human diseases are caused because of excess acid values in body. "Dr. Otto Warburg" who was a Nobel Prize winner for his significant research in blood pH & disease relation has stated that, "NO DISEASE

INCLUDING CANCER CAN EXIST IN ALKALINE ENVIRONMENT".

Acid in blood directly affects mainly three systems which are:

1. Brain & Nervous System
2. Blood Vessels
3. Cell

When excess acid strikes brain, it directly alters many neurochemical reactions & may cause neurological disorders like meningitis, neuromuscular dystrophy, seizures or altered behaviors. When this acid encounters with our cardiovascular system, arteriosclerosis, atherosclerosis or rupturing of small blood vessels may happen. Third system, which got influenced adversely by excess acid, is cell & tissue functioning skin disorders or even cancer is caused by excess acid in body. Excess acid promotes every bio-chemical reaction abnormally fast, including cell division and uncontrolled over division of cells is known as cancer.

These days, it is very tough to avoid excess acid from entering our body because our modern food culture is majorly acid forming. Let's start from soft drink which has pH like strong acids (pH of 2.5), every crop is being sprayed with insecticides and other chemicals resulting acid in our food plate. From refined cooking oil to biscuits, pasteurized milk to processed cheese, our snacks & even drinking water we managed to add acid contents almost in everything we consume. That's why I always say that our today's modern society is going through dark ages of food and health.

Chapter – 2 Loud & False: The Cholesterol

In last few decades, the loudly & widely spread misconception or we can say a most decorated lie is the cholesterol. Cholesterol is getting popular in todays' world for all the wrong reasons as cholesterols are seen in a parallel line with heart diseases & vascular disorders. Most of the medical media, famous medical journals, health organizations are presenting cholesterol as a culprit for deaths related to cardio-vascular disorders. But, there is a story which is being buried underground for some mean reasons. In very starting of this medical revolution era, normal value of cholesterols were assumed to be approximately 300 but this number was declared false by a panel of doctors & now, the ideal value of blood cholesterol is around 200. This shift has given birth to a very big industry designed to keep cholesterol level as less as possible. Overnight a million & trillion-dollar industry stands up which is selling you anti-cholesterol tablets, anti-cholesterol dietary supplements, refined oil with chemical inside it but a photo of smiling heart posted on the bottle. This lie was so loud that everyone opted for these toxic shifts believing that their conventional oils, ghee & other healthy source of fat are danger for their lives.

A very big section of our society starts consuming these refined & chemical added oils in their diet. Some corporate doctors were getting paid for promoting this lie & I must say they perform their duty very well. Even today, majority of highly trained (not educated) doctors from very big institutes are maintaining the legacy of promoting such unnatural & chemical added eatables as a health symbol.

To understand more about this cholesterol myth, we look from where all this biased information is coming. Let's assume, if there is a case of fire accident somewhere, which is getting uncontrolled. The firefighter department will reach that area & they will try to get control over the fire. Though firefighters were present at the place of fire but they cannot be counted or considered as a factor of causing fire accident but if a patient gets heart attack and cholesterol is found inside that blood vessel, does not prove cholesterol as attack agents. The function of LDL (Low density lipoprotein) is to repair the internal lining of blood vessels. If the damage to the internal lining of those blood vessels is high, more & more LDL will be sent at that place for repair purpose but we have forgotten this basic physiological process and messed this issue very badly. Instead of looking at those factors we are just lost in this cholesterol & heart disease theory.

Let's assume, if a person is kept on zero fat diet for a long period though it is impossible but still to make my point clear I need to bring this hypothetical example before you. A person who is kept on fat free diet can never have zero cholesterol in his blood. So do you really think that all the cholesterol in your body is coming from a fatty diet? In fact, the truth is very different from what you know approximately 70 percent of the cholesterol is made independently by your body, irrespective of what you eat. Only 30 percent of the total cholesterol in your body is contributed by dietary factors. So what does it mean? If cholesterol is really a bad guy then why your body is making it continuously in such a huge amount. Fact is, Cholesterols are needed to make various hormones, tissue repair, cell repair, nerve conduction, skin, brain cells. All major sex hormones need cholesterols as raw material. On the whole, it could be said that life can't survive without Cholesterols. So, this anti-cholesterol movement is a foolish idea. In fact, there are number of evidences in latest research papers from leading universities worldwide, especially in U.S.A. Which reveals that fat free diet is causing more damage & anti-cholesterol medication are linked directly to increased incidents of heart attack. Don't only trust my words go & search by your own, this whole information is just one Google search away from you.

Let me put a light on one more factor regarding cholesterol which may give you a feel as you are fooled by this medical industry. I want you to imagine the picture of a cholesterol molecule & observe how this molecule looks to you. Is it a small ball or mini droplet of fat? If yes, then please look at the name of cholesterol once again. In medical term, we call it lipoprotein; can you see that word protein in it?

Yes, it is a type of protein which is bonded to a small fat molecule. Now rethink what the advertisements are telling you as cholesterol causing factors. In very simple words for your understanding, I would say that cholesterol is a protein riding on a fat vehicle for its transportation. One more misconception which you must have familiar with, is the way they present you those two types of cholesterol. First is HDL (high density lipoproteins) which is called good cholesterol and second is LDL (low density lipoproteins) which is Bad Cholesterol in their perception. Which I believe is the worst way to explain both of them. Science recognizes both of them as just cholesterols; having different densities and hence different functions. Both of them are needed in body to perform their respective functions. Body never produces anything by its own, which is bad for you. Medical professionals who are making such good & bad classifications should respect body and its physiological process. They might not be aware of the use & importance of everything that the body is producing for its survival and wellbeing.

Anti-Cholesterol Medicines and Blood Thinners: In last few decades, number one selling drugs worldwide is antihypertensive, anti-cholesterol, blood thinners and anti-diabetes. Especially, if we talk about anti-cholesterol medicine and blood-thinner these two drugs are crowned as lifesaving drugs but actually, these drugs are causing more deaths rather than high cholesterol levels. Statins (drug used as anti-cholesterol) are being prescribed worldwide as a miraculous drug to fight against heart diseases but the damage this medicine has given to mankind is irreversible and ruthless. Before we start, it is important to discuss that how these anti-cholesterol tablets works. Statin interferes in the chain of process by which cholesterols are made in body. When this chain is broken, it is not only cholesterol synthesis which is being affected adversely but many other vital byproducts on which our body & specially heart rely upon. One of them is co-enzyme Q-10 which is very powerful enzyme and gives support to many vital organs especially heart. Once statin drugs interfere in this chain reaction many important enzymes, co-factors, cholesterols and other necessary byproducts got blocked. So, it means not only cholesterols are blocked with statins but vital co-enzyme Q-10 is also not synthesized which makes the risk 100 times bigger. Because, on one hand, we are blocking the benefits & functions of cholesterol in the body & on other hand, we are also hampering co-enzyme Q-10 to protect our heart from the damage caused by decreasing cholesterol level in blood. Anti-cholesterol medicine damages every system of our body specially those who needs cholesterol in priority for their working. In U.S., Alzheimer is the biggest epidemic in senior citizen & it is not because of their genetic code or idiopathic but in fact, it is a side effect of anti-cholesterol medicines. U.S. is the largest consumer of anti-cholesterol medicines & metabolic disorder related medications. India is also on the way to get in trap of Alzheimer & other mental health issues. In next 10 years, we will witness a sudden burst of this disease & our modern medicine system will add some more fancy tablets to the bags of such patients but, it will be all in vain. I am sorry to say this but, being a responsible physician of this nation it is my moral duty to emphasis on the health related warning signs.

Sexual disorder, loss of libido, infertility, premature aging is all the gift of this low fat stigma, because our reproductive system needs mainly cholesterols & lipids as a raw material for all its functions.

Brain is an organ which is made up of approximately 50 percent of cholesterol. If we take anti-cholesterol medicine for regular basis the brain will punish you back in the form of stress, depression, epilepsy, mania, Alzheimer & other neurological conditions.

You could be shocked to know that anti-cholesterol medicines are also a cause of heart-attack. Yes, you heard it right. Ask yourself, does these anti-cholesterol medicines are worth or serving its purpose? Actually! it is putting your heart at risk but it is being advertised as cardio-protective, heart friendly and as a safe-guard from heart-attacks; God Bless Modern Medicine. In this whole story, most shocking thing for me is that these drugs are being prescribed by those doctors who believe for themselves as they are specialists of heart and their study teaches them to treat, protect and strengthens the heart. Somehow, when your body tries to bear this damage they don't stop here, now they will also give you a blood thinner as a complementary thing to enhance your self-destruction process. We don't have to be a rocket scientist to imagine what it means to dilute your blood; no one even likes their tea, coffee or fruit juice to be diluted with water and these guys are telling you to dilute your blood on daily basis with a chemical tablet. I think while prescribing such drugs, they are somewhere forgetting or ignoring the benefits and role of blood in body. A thin blood can damage you in many ways but here I will explain the damage of blood thinners only on heart. Your heart is a muscle and it is such an extra-ordinary muscle which has to work continuously from the day you born till the day you will die. There is no other muscle except heart which can work continuously without a break for even a minute. Imagine, if you have to move your bicep continuously for only an hour. Your bicep muscle will be damaged permanently but your heart is working regularly from years and is committed to do the same till your last breath. For such an extraordinary work your heart needs only good quality of blood and in good quantity. But some idiots are telling you to dilute your blood daily for the sake of your heart. I have no words to praise their advanced understanding towards human body and their expertise in treating diseases related to heart.

Your Clueless Cardiologist:

This whole model of modern medicine is designed to act against basic physiology of body. Other drawbacks in this system is, doctor of one system doesn't know exactly that what is the link of heart with other organs nor they are aware of what damage will their medicine can throw on other systems of the body. When a cardiologist is prescribing an anti-cholesterol medicine to his patient with raised cholesterol levels, he is unaware that this medicine will damage brain, nervous system, immunity & eventually heart itself.

Now let me explain why I called them clueless. A patient name John visited his doctor's office for routine checkup. Doctor finds that John is having raised cholesterol level in his blood investigation report. After seeing this report, while doctor was prescribing anti-cholesterol medicine to John, he asked doctor, "Doctor are you really very sure that this cholesterol is raised in my body for all the evil causes & dragging me towards a serious heart problem. Being a biology professor I know 50 percent of our body needs cholesterol for daily routine working. My brain, nervous system, cortisol, sex hormones, skin, certain portions of eye, some internal visceral organs, neurotransmitters, fluid inside my joints & many more essential body parts either are made up of cholesterol or needs cholesterol for normal working & repair. Sir, can you please clear my doubt that on what grounds you are so sure that this cholesterol is not raised in my body for repair of any organ or there is any need of some extra cholesterol to deal with stress or it's not raised for temporary basis as my body is preparing to compensate hormonal need because cholesterol are the raw material of many essential hormones". After hearing this John's doctor was speechless and clueless. But, this silence of John's doctor speaks very loudly. I have just one simple question & I leave it up to you that what you think & what you believe. There are approximately nine (9) million creatures in animal kingdom on this planet. Except humans, no other creature depends on chemical added tablets or any other form of modern medicine to fix their health issues but humans having so called developed health care system; is suffering from the diseases which were never been even existed on this planet. Daily our health statics is falling down and this destruction is not stopping. Whom to Blame for all this?

Remedying Heart Diseases:

One basic thing which is often ignored is that, any symptom produced in your body indicates some kind of disorder. But trying to suppress only symptoms without finding its cause is not a good idea. Today, most of the problems that our world is facing are either caused by our faulty eating habits & life style or by wrong kind of treatment we use for any minor or major health issue. As far as heart is concerned, we just need very healthy quality of blood which will come from our healthy diet because as a continuously working muscle, our heart needs huge amount of nutrients through blood to work efficiently. This is the reason our body is designed in a way that a significant amount of blood is being provided to heart through coronary artery. This is the only organ receiving such a huge quantity of blood for its nutrition. No such organ receives this much amount of blood, a direct division from aorta is supplied for the nutrition of heart alone, which we know as coronary artery. The design of our heart and this kind of arrangement for blood is revealing the entire story, that what is the importance of healthy supply of blood towards heart. A healthy heart needs good diet, proper blood supply, sufficient amount of oxygen in blood, proper exercise & sleep. Any kind of heart diseases will be caused if any one or more from above mentioned factors is interrupted. Unfortunately, our modern medical system is telling us as if heart disease is deficiency of some tablets that could be blood thinner, statins, anti-hypertensive or ACE inhibitors. They are not talking about nutrients, trace minerals, essential amino-acids and proper blood supply.

After nutrition, second important thing your heart will require to work efficiently is exercise. Because when you exercise the exchange of blood through heart also increases. Exercise promote more & more blood to run through heart & hence availing extra nutrition (carried in blood) to heart resulting your heart will work as an honest worker for you. This could be started with gentle jumping & jogging as per the stamina & capability of your body. Subsequently, this could be increased with time from jogging to jumping & then gradually preparing for running. Believe me your heart does not needs any chemical base tablet to work efficiently.

Look at the animals, can you ever see a tiger taking anti-cholesterol medicine as he eats only red meat & he has to keep his heart healthy for long running. Do you believe elephant being so huge &

fatty needs blood thinner to avoid blocking & cardiac attacks because of cholesterols? In fact, if you start giving these so-called lifesaving anti-cholesterol medicines & blood thinners to any animal, it will firstly affect their health & finally a life threating condition may develop in them. This whole medical industry is being driven by big pharmaceutical companies, who are not concerned or responsible for your health; they are only concerned with their sales value & making every possible effort to increase their sales day by day. Pharmaceutical companies are hiding themselves because they are not using their own mouth to say this. Some doctors are selling this lie & medicines both for them.

Chapter – 3
High Blood Pressure

Hypertension is most common and still least known health condition. This is a condition, when your blood pressure is raised from normal level. But there is very dissimilarities regarding the normal levels of blood pressure. In some countries, a systolic pressure of 110 mm/Hg is considered normal while in some other countries 140 mm/Hg systolic pressure is considered normal. In India & many other countries normal value for blood pressure is 120/80 mm/Hg. But enforcing one number for different individuals is unfair in my opinion. Everyone is unique; everybody has their own unique configuration, so it is obvious that normal value of blood pressure may vary from person to person. But our medical system is designed to work on numbers without looking at physiological reasons, geographical area & other factors, which may affect blood pressure.

One thing we must know about blood pressure is that it is adaptive. Which means this pressure adapts or varies as per the requirement of body. High blood pressure is not a disease in itself. But it is an indication that something went wrong with the physiology of body. So what do you expect from your doctor, when you visits your doctor's office with high blood pressure. The doctor must try to investigate the reason for high blood pressure &

give you solutions for the cause not for the symptoms but unfortunately, he will only prescribe you some anti-hypertensive medicine which is dangerous and also an idiotic action.

In my clinical practice, I often talk to patients who are taking anti-hypertensive tablets from years because their doctor told him to do so. Neither patient nor his doctor have an idea why this pressure is consistently high & what damage these anti-hypertensive medicines are doing to them. Let's assume, a patient with renal dysfunction & hypertension, consulting his doctor. What his doctor will explain him, "Your high blood pressure has damaged your kidneys" & the patient will be prescribed high grade anti-hypertensive medicines. But this approach is totally against the flow of the body. If any portion or organ of your body got damaged, your body will try to throw more & more blood towards that area to ensure proper & speedy recovery. If we are just trying to pull down blood pressure without addressing the root cause it will give an irreparable loss to the body. There are some conditions, when your blood pressure needs to be high but ignorance of our modern medical system has created a mess. Even if you are sleeping, sitting, standing, walking, running or eating you may have certain effect on your blood pressure. But if this blood pressure is markedly raised for long period; reason must be big. Only prescribing some fancy names of tablets for dropping down blood pressure forcefully is a sign of a robotic doctor who is not capable of understanding body & its disorders. What will happen, if a person is having his normal blood pressure 150/90 mm/Hg & his doctor prescribes him some medicines to bring it down up to 120/80 mm/Hg which is considered normal. Such actions are really damaging to the body, because body always act very smart and all the changes made by the body is for its survival or recovery. I admit that having high blood pressure is even more dangerous. Before grabbing pen and immediately starts writing some fancy branded tablets, doctors must rethink for the sake of their studies to at least try once and investigate for the cause. So, if there is no definite number for normal blood pressure then what is the right method or criteria for a blood pressure to be considered normal?

A practitioner must look at the difference between systolic & diastolic pressure & it must be ideally 40. Which means a pressure of 120/80 mm/Hg having difference of 40 should be considered normal. Similarly 130/90, 140/100 is also normal as the difference between systolic & diastolic is maintained at 40. Change in this difference needs your special attention or we might think of other risks.

Categories of Blood Pressure:

Hypertension is divided into three stages depending upon its value. Systolic pressure of 130-139 is considered as stage 1 hypertension, Systolic pressure of 140-149 is considered as a stage 2 hypertension & Systolic pressure of 180 or more is called hypertensive crisis. But before classifying hypertension into these stages, we must categories hypertension into two categories first is dependent

& second is non-dependent (which is my own way of classifying this).

Dependent Hypertension:

This is actually a primary kind of hypertension which is caused by some basic factors; such cases will only develop hypertension by some temporary factors like constipation, sleeplessness, travelling, unhealthy food or stress. This is not permanent & will be dependent on the factor for hypertension as we remove that factor, blood pressure will be normal. This is primary type of hypertension & usually it doesn't indicate any bigger physiological damage in the body. If that, patient is given healthy food, proper sleep, stress free environment & ensuring for his/her proper bowl clearance daily, the raised blood pressure of that patient will be normal without any medication.

Note:

Sometimes calcium deficiency also causes tachycardia & high blood pressure. This is also considered as a dependent hypertension.

Non-Dependent Hypertension:

This kind of hypertension has nothing to do with your bowl habit or mental status. This type of blood pressure will be consistently high. Such hypertension needs proper diagnosis, as it indicates some significant physiological change due to some sort of pathology or damage, because of toxicity. This kind of hypertension will never go by its own unless root cause is addressed. In general 3 out of 10 patients fall under this category.

Salt & Hypertension:

Almost everybody is familiar with the role of salt in causing hypertension. So, there are many doctors who are prescribing salt free diet for their patients to help them in hypertension. This might be helpful, if it is prescribed once in a week or twice a month but if anyone follows more than prescribed, this could lead to dangerous or even fatal results because among all the nutrients & minerals: Sodium is most important mineral in the body from muscle contraction to Nervous conduction. It is needed within the cell, outside the cell or we can say, sodium is required in almost all minor & major action of the body. Common salt which we use is NaCl. This NaCl disperses into two molecules which are sodium (Na) and chlorine (Cl). Sodium has its requirement in almost every vital process of the body. Similarly, chlorine from this salt is also required in various actions of cell and body. Chlorine has direct impact on our digestive system. Chlorine molecule from Sodium Chloride (NaCl) is used to produce acid of our stomach which is HCl. Without HCl, proteins & fats in the diet could not be broken & digested, which is a serious issue.

So, from above discussion, it is clear that opting salt free diet for regular basis is not a good idea but the table salt or sea salt has its own danger. NaCl should also be added in our diet in diluted form because sodium molecule (Na) needs a parallel molecule to balance its actions & that molecule is Potassium (K). Potassium is very crucial element which is needed in very huge amount by our body on daily basis. This sodium and potassium molecule works in a line to perform various significant actions within the body. We in our medical language, refer it as sodium potassium pump. Sodium without presence of potassium is a killer molecule. Normal saline (NS) which is administrated intravenously to the patients in hospital has its concentration of NS 0.09 percent which is very extensively diluted form. Imagine, if this concentration is raised above 50 percent & than given intravenously (IV) to the patient, he can die within seconds by arrest of all voluntary & involuntary muscles. So, from this long salt story what point we raised?

Salt is important for our body but not in concentrated and isolated form. Sea salts & table salts are 100 percent pure NaCl molecule, whereas, the salt like rock salt & Celtic salt are natural salts having 70 percent NaCl molecule & 30 percent fortified minerals like potassium, magnesium, iron & others. That's why sea salt should never be used in cooking as it is slow poison where as other natural salts are beneficial in numerous ways & boon to humanity.

Moreover, as I always insist to look at the nature what it wants you to do. Your body is a spec of this universe and has a beautiful collaboration. Everything regarding health needs not a million-dollar research. Just be sensitive enough to feel the message of nature. Concerning salt, your body will clearly say you how the salt is required. The message from your body is loud and clear enough; you cannot have any meal without salt as your taste buds will reject it. Similarly, minor over-dose of salt also tastes bitter, like some kind of poison. In addition, you cannot eat one tablespoon of salt directly, through the mouth.

This is clear message from your body that salt is necessary in your meal but neither in a heavy-dose nor in a concentrated form.

Just respect the nature and this beautiful creation of nature, what we refer as a human body. It will signal you all in a strong way that what is healthy and what is not. The only problem with us is we are not sensitive enough to listen.

Natural Beta Blockers:

The most famous and effective category of drugs used in hypertension is beta-blockers. Beta-Blockers are used in almost every country for management of high blood pressure. These drugs when used regularly produce some side effects which damages our muscles of heart & other systems also. Besides all the side-effects to the consumers, these pharmaceutical companies are yielding trillion-dollar profit per day & also risking our lives. Whereas, there are different types of natural beta-blockers which are not only capable of controlling hypertension but also benefits in numerous other ways. Magnesium is one of such a leading element which works as natural beta-blocker in our body and also boosts immunity. All the dark green vegetables and leafy vegetables are rich source of magnesium, including these stuff in diet on a regular basis will be a gift to your body.

Second molecule, which controls increased heart rate & thus helps to control hypertension, is calcium. Many vegetables, fruits & butter are good source of natural calcium. The calcium tablets which you are getting from health stores are not that calcium which is required in your body. These tablets are not free & isolated calcium molecule. They are calcium carbonate (CaCo3) tablets, which is lime stone. Instead of paying for calcium carbonate, it is better to chew lime stone either. So, it is not advisable to consume either calcium tablets or lime stone for the sake of calcium because your body is not going to use this inferior type of calcium. If you want to consume calcium as a supplement for health reasons you must consult a qualified Ayurvedic physician and ask him for natural source of calcium because Ayurveda is the only pathy which offers some of the best sources for calcium in medicinal form e.g. Mukta Pishti (made form pearl), Parvaal Pishti (made from coral & many more). These kinds of calcium will help in controlling tachycardia, reducing heat element from the body & most of the hypertension patients could be benefitted from only such kind of natural calcium.

Responsive Hypertension:

This kind of hypertension is developed in body because of stress response. There are mainly three kinds of stress to our body, which are physical, chemical & emotional stress. Body responds in very same manner in response to any kind of stress. Which means your body cannot differentiate between these three types of stress. Body follows a standard protocol to deal with stress. First thing your body perceives regarding stress is, as it's an emergency situation. This activates adrenal glands & a strong anti-inflammatory, steroidal hormone is released from cortex of adrenal glands known as cortisol. This cortisol aligns the body in a very protective manner as a shield against stress. Various changes which body made under the effect of cortisol are meant to deal with all the three types of stress at the same time. One of the major changes is increasing blood pressure and blood cholesterol levels. But, what allopathic doctor will see is only raised cholesterol and blood pressure. They have nothing to do with those three kinds of stress. But unless exact cause is diagnosed and necessary actions are taken, hypertension could be suppressed with some allopathic tablets.

Physical, Chemical & Emotional Stress:

Physical Stress:

Let's assume a person has physical stress because of some kind of internal organ damage like liver, kidney or large intestine. Even a past surgery can contribute to a physical stress in your today's life. Which means a person may carry stress of the surgery in his body even after years from surgery. This is the reason, why some patients develop hypertension or gain weight after surgical procedure. This kind of hypertension is often seen when we have to rejuvenate or heal the portion of the body carrying physical stress. Untreated pain like knee pain or low back pain if suppressed with pain-killers or NSAID's also results in hypertension because pain also generates stress response in the body. Unless that portion is rejuvenated, body will keep behaving as a carrier of stress.

Chemical Stress:

Chemical stress will only occur in body when any artificial molecule enters our system. Higher the number of chemical stress agents; higher will be the stress level in the body. These artificial molecules are everywhere in today's world that's why we see number of patients under chemical stress or oxidative stress so frequently. Some of the diseases related to chemical stress are respiratory disorders, allergies, skin irritations, chronic inflammation, multiple-sclerosis, internal organ damage like liver, kidney or heart, hypertension and many more. Chemical stress is also a leading cause of auto-immune disorders.

So, if the list of diseases related to chemical stress is so long, we have to be aware that from where all this chemical is entering in our body? Refined oil, fried food, adulteration in food, chemical like chlorine is added in drinking water, all skin care products which have harmful chemicals in it like methyl paraben & other harmful chemicals which is even tough to pronounce & more tougher to throw out from the body, different types of deodorants or perfumes which we inhale daily. All of above comes under the category of chemical stress causing factors. In recent years, even vegetables, commercially produced dairy products & commercially raised animals also falls in this category. Detoxification is the best way to deal with any diseases related to chemical stress.

Emotional Stress:

Emotional stress is basically a situation which affects your emotional values or sentiments. Having bad social reputation, loss of loved one, habit of excessive thinking, keeping higher expectations without acting or working to achieve that, reading vulgar literature or watching porn, multiple love affairs at same time, laziness in profession & personal life, getting up late in the morning are prime causes for emotional stress. Good quality of counseling and motivation, high quality literature or changing surrounding atmosphere completely usually helps the patients high emotional stress level or hypertension related to it.

Chapter – 4
Ruthless Nail and Hammer Method

The fundamental mistake in our modern medical system is this whole industry is designed to suppress only symptoms by completely ignoring the cause. Though, I believe allopathic medicinal system has invented many miraculous medicines which aids to humanity and suppresses the suffering. I also believe painkiller is one of the greatest inventions and it is serving its cause very well. Biggest fear and torturing thing for human body is pain. No one wants to bear pain even for a while, but the only issue with painkiller is, it has nothing to do with the cause. Use of painkiller in emergency condition is like a boon but when these painkillers are thrown ignorantly over lifestyle disorders; then, it creates havoc.

Pain is like an indication that something went wrong with the functioning of the body or that particular body part. Pain is an expression of body to drag your immediate attention towards that area but when you use only painkiller without investigating the cause you are refusing to hear your body's message. While driving a car, if your car's meter shows alarming lights and sound (beep) what will you do? Will you visit nearest service station for checkup and find out the problem or you will just cut the wire to turn off warning signs. Cutting wire is same as we are dealing with pains by use of painkillers. Suppose your knee joint is hurting because of some functional disorder, it should be understood that your knee joint wants you to restrict movement and look for the cause and solution but when you visit your doctor he will give you some painkillers, some calcium tablets or multivitamins. In most extreme cases, doctor may advise you some steroids also. Within a couple of minutes to an hour, you can successfully suppress your pain and restores the movement of the joint normally. This is an act against your body because the joint which was demanding rest will be now moved forcefully and damaged more.

Listening any symptoms from patient and immediately prescribing medicines to suppress that symptom without giving time to think, investigate and trying to address the root cause is not a healthy health care system. This style of practicing medicines is not the job of any qualified doctor. Doctors should leave such cheap style of practicing for unregistered and unqualified doctors or illegal pharmacists who behaves like a doctor in their respective areas. Qualified doctors must show some respect to human body and their study as well, in the form of a holistic healing diet regimen and some life style advises to heal their patients. But the bitter truth is most of the medicines in allopathic system is actually causing that diseases for which those medicines are designed to heal. Can you imagine what does it mean? We really need to improve our healthcare system, otherwise in next 50 years consequences will be horrifying. Let's understand this more with some examples and fact base discussion.

Inflammation and NSAID's:

Non-steroidal anti-inflammatory drugs (NSAID) are a family of drugs which are used for inflammatory disorders and pain. Before moving further, let's try to understand what inflammation is and why it is caused. Inflammation is a broad topic that's why an independent chapter is given in this book only on inflammation. Inflammation is actually a healing or defense mechanism of your body. If any portion of the body gets injured, body supplies some extra blood to that portion to ensure extra-nutrition and healing, in an addition, temperature is also raised slightly in that area to make the healing process fast. But anti-inflammatory drugs hinder this process, resulting in a prolonged unhealed area or an organ. In diseases like osteoarthritis, rheumatoid arthritis, cervical or lumber spondylitis, medical doctors advise anti-inflammatory drug to be taken regularly. Patients also get relief from the first dose and this will go for some months or years but finally when that portion is damaged beyond a level, the joint is now in an untreatable condition because regular painkillers has damaged the joint and body in many ways and also increased inflammation by many folds. So, the industry captures you by starting with a painkiller for joint pain which will eventually end at total knee replacement surgery.

Mental Health and SSRI:

Selective Serotonin Reuptake Inhibitor (SSRI) which is mainly used for depression, anxiety and other mental disorder. In modern medicine, exact action mechanism of SSRI is still unknown to them but it is used in many psychological disorders. It suppresses certain centers of brain, by inhibiting the working of brain. But side effects of these drugs are again severe mental disorders, behavior disorders, even suicidal tendencies and these adverse effects are not my assumptions, this is what their research tells us. What kind of health care system we have developed is a matter of great shame. Our brain is an organ which requires ketone bodies (which come from fat) Glucose (which come from different sources), sufficient amount of oxygen and some essential form of amino acids. Most of the mental disorder is basically the result of certain deficiencies but nobody is going to tell you this or try to look at the nutritional aspect in mental disorder. I must say, race of inventing newer medicines has pushed out physiology of body from the minds of doctors now they are just sensitive to symptoms and has expertise to choose a relevant tablet immediately as they listens any symptom.

Gastritis and Ant-Acids:

Hyperacidity or heart burn is caused due to excess of acids in stomach is a biggest lie we have been informed. This concept is so weekly understood by our modern world that even simple indigestion or hyperacidity is a lifelong disorder now and doctors are advising their patients to take these medicines daily. Not only this, they also advice if a type of ant-acid named 'proton pump inhibitor' is taken empty stomach daily your digestion will be benefitted and promoted. They literally believe that ant-acids are safe to be consumed regularly.

But my curiosity is how they are successful to convince people for a simple gastric trouble to be medicated daily for its better functioning. Fact is, long term use of ant-acids cause many health issues including severe gastritis itself. Let's look at the science now, in your whole digestive system stomach is the only organ which should be acidic because this acid will break your food, kills pathogen in food and emulsifies the fat present in food. This acid is highly strong in healthy and young person but with age this acid becomes weak and digestion also starts retarding. The pH of stomach should be less than 2 which mean this acid can dissolves the bones also. This acid is not supposed to come up in the food pipe unless this acid becomes weaker or diluted. Because at the upper end of stomach and base of food pipe (junction of food pipe and stomach) there is a sphincter or in simple words you can say a barrier which stops stomach acid from popping up into food pipe. This sphincter works only when there is acid in stomach. Rest of the time, this sphincter remains relaxed which means this sphincter works on the acid strength of stomach. Stronger the acid, tighter will be the sphincter and weak acid relaxes this sphincter resulting, stomach acid get a chance to seep out from this sphincter into esophagus. Internal lining of esophagus (food pipe) is not protected from acid by any extra protective layer. This acid causes the burning sensation in food pipe, which is felt in the middle of the chest at the level of the heart. That's why it is also known as heart burn. These ant-acids makes weak acid even weaker or almost neutral to suppress heart burn but this is very dangerous even beyond your imagination. The safest drug you know as ant-acids can develop anything from weak immunity to even mental disorders, let's see how.

Nutrition of body is not dependent on what we eat but it is what we have digested; taking ant-acid tablet will collapse your digestion specially digestion of fat because fat needs strong acid to be broken for digestion and absorption. Deficiency of fatty acids and fat soluble vitamins (vitamin A, D, E and K) causing infertility, pre-mature aging, weak bones, sexual weakness, hormone disturbance in females, dull skin, hair fall, fatigue, restless leg syndrome , vision problems and many more related disorders because all the above mentioned diseases or symptoms needs either fat soluble vitamins or fatty acid for their functioning but ant-acid had destroyed that fat metabolism path.

Instead of treating gastritis or hyperacidity with ant-acid tablets if doctors try to give some probiotic drinks like “Kombucha tea”, artificial enzymes to enhance digestion or many herbal solution as in Indian Ayurvedic medicine system or Chinese herbs therapy; the health status of society will be definitely better than today. Ant-acids not only kill acid of stomach but it affects whole body because each and every system is dependent on digestion.

There is a famous health saying which says, "We are what we eat" but even this not true in my opinion. Actually, "We are what we have digested." By the way, hyperacidity is technically wrong name given to this condition and I believe this name had confused many innocent doctors as this name sounds like disorder of excess acid. I suggest and coin the term W.A.S. for this condition which is “Weak Acid Syndrome” and this name will justify with the condition perfectly. May be this could change the perception of doctors towards this condition as well.

General Weakness and Multivitamins:

One more famous myth in medical world is regarding multivitamins not even a single book in medical schools or colleges tells that vitamins are the unit of energy in body, but doctors are continuously linking energy with vitamins. Energy unit of body is "pyruvate" which is synthesized inside the cell after series of reaction also known as "Kreb Cycle". Vitamins are undoubtedly vital for body but they only helps in proper functioning of body & act as a factor in many chemical reactions. Here are mainly two points which should be brought under notice:-

1. Without knowing which vitamin is deficient in the body, how we can use a commercially designed multivitamin tablet or capsule which is claimed to be a complete package of all the required nutrients. Some people may argue that taking multivitamins in tablets is healthy & if it

is not healthy; at least, it is safe but this is also not true. Regular intake of multivitamins creates an addiction for constant multivitamins; simultaneously, it also suppresses the absorption & synthesis of natural vitamins in the body. Multivitamins which were designed to keep you healthy & energetic are actually depleting natural reserve & synthesis of these vitamins in the body.

2. Artificial Vitamins used in Multivitamin Capsule & tablets are actually derived as a petroleum product, which is toxic in nature & neither your body accepts it nor uses it. After taking such multivitamin, you can find this multivitamin in urine. Urine will shows yellow color & even slight smell of these multivitamins, which is a proof that your body has rejected your artificial multivitamin. Expensive urine is the only benefit which you can have from such multivitamins. Healthy diet, proper digestion, fresh air & reasonable amount of workout are the only authentic natural multivitamin package you can have.

Tip:

To ensure proper nutrients in your body we must focus on absorbing maximum nutrients from the food we eat because weak digestion and absorption throws out many nutrients from the body with fecal matter. Chewing the food well increases the surface area of your food and helps body to digest and absorb well. In this fast paced lifestyle, this fundamental rule is ignored very badly. Chewing the food is only natural kind of digestive tonic and multivitamin you can have.

High Blood pressure & Anti- hypertensive Medicines:

Today, every 6 out of 10 adult person in our world are suffering from hypertension, being so common, it is still least understood. On the name of treatment what your doctor offers you is some kind of tablets which belongs to Beta-blocker, nitrates, calcium channel blocker, ACE inhibitor or in some cases diuretics or mild sedatives. We are advised to take these medicines daily for the sake of good health. But actually these medicines are very harmful, if they are taken on regular basis. When you visit your doctor's office with high blood pressure, he will check your blood pressure & hand over you some tablets to lower it. He will never try to find the cause and try to fix it because of his ignorance & these medicines will cause damage to your cardiovascular system, resulting in serious health issue within few years & if ask for the reason, they will not admit their ignorance but try to convince you that taking these medicines is absolutely normal & safer as well.

Hypertension is not a lifelong condition; it could be cured permanently by looking at its cause rather than engulfing some tablets. 50-60 percent of hypertension cases could be cured permanently within few weeks but our approach towards diseases should be improved. Not only hypertension or mental disorder almost every disease is getting worsened with the treatment being offered to us by this allopathic system of medicine. Metformin is a tablet used in Type-II diabetes but this tablet is the leading cause for various diabetic complications and especially insulin resistance.

Allopurinol is a tablet which is used in gout but this tablet contributes to increase inflammatory reactions in body resulting in more severe form of gout & joint degeneration. Other side-effect includes joint pain, unusual bleeding, urine disorder, burning sensation and even worsening gout symptoms. This tablet also damages kidney & liver, in addition to the joints. Is this really a developed medicinal system for which we are tapping our back & being proud of?

Bacterial Infections & Antibiotic Use:

Though, I believe use of antibiotics in some serious conditions is highly beneficial and lifesaving but the reason behind these bacterial infections is completely ignored. We all know, human body is a carrier of millions and millions of bacteria. On an average human body, total bacterial count is more than the total population of humans on this planet Earth. But, these bacteria do not harm us; in fact, they are vital for our healthy skin and healthy gut. We call them good bacteria or friendly bacteria. So, what makes any bacteria bad for us?

Our Modern Science has messed this topic again by their analytic & superficial approach. What they assume is that it is the bacteria which are causing infection in the body but it isn't true again.

Look at the nature, where these bad bacteria, maggots etc. germinate? It always germinates on dead and decaying stuff. Similarly, bacteria can only attack on the dead cells of our body. No Bacteria is powerful enough to attack human body, this is very funny to me. How can they even imagine that an under developed organism which is not visible even to our naked eyes can do harm to such an evolved creature of this planet. Logically, higher bacterial infection does not mean Bad bacteria are growing inside body, it simply means by some reasons cells insides the body are dying. Rather than focusing on higher & higher class of antibiotics we must focus on the fact that what's wrong with the body that body is caring so many dead cells. It is not a sin to use antibiotics. We must use them, if we have invented them but using only and only antibiotics by completely ignoring the cause of cell death is silly. Look at the person after death, his body will start decaying after few hours of death. This is how mother-nature works. Everything which is dead has to be eaten up by bacteria and they are designed to do so. Job of bacteria is to clean the garbage of this planet. Biological garbage is the main food of bacteria. So next time, whenever you look at bacterial infection I expect you to look that infection with a logical approach this time.

No doctor in this world can explain you the cause of bacterial infection. They can only tell you how to kill these bacteria.

I am not saying that Allopathic doctors are lying to you. No, not at all, 80 percent of doctors are genuine and nice. But it’s the pharmaceutical companies which are lying to them.

Who is actually responsible for this?

It is not actually 100 percent fault of allopathic doctor. No doctor in this world wants to hurt their patients, if they have any other safer option. Similarly, allopathic doctors are not practicing in a flaw full manner with some kind of bad deeds in their minds. They are bounded to do such practice because it is all what they have been taught. They don't know or more correctly I can say, they can't perceive that the disease which they are treating with heavy steroids or anti-inflammatory

Drugs could be fixed in a safer & beneficial way. They are trained only in this way to react and act on symptoms only.

Now let's move backwards to medical colleges. Is there any fault with the studies or syllabus? It is also a non-considerable point. Because, before teaching them medicines, they are taught detailed knowledge of anatomy, physiology & bio-chemistry. They know almost everything what I discussed majorly in this book, because even I acquired all these concepts & my understanding towards human body from these above maintained three subjects. "Guyton", which is considered as a "Bible" in human physiology speaks very clearly the benefits of fats, effect of fat on insulin response and almost everything regarding human body working and cause of diseases. In fact, in pharmacology, the list of side-effects from any allopathic medicine is longer than their benefits. So, if doctors are not responsible for all this; their study is complete and authentic; then from where this all stuff is coming from.

According to my perception, a student enters in a medical college with a golden heart & a passion to serve the humanity. This is a true fact, no-one can deny from this. But, the gap between medical college & professional life changes the game. In medical colleges, medical science is taught & followed but in medical practice this science is vanished or fades up & everything runs on medical culture & profit industry. This medical culture is very different from medical science. I am a strong follower of medical science, but this medical culture is actually cruel. Let me make my point more transparent here, medical science will tell you to go for the reason of any diseases, says high blood pressure, but medical culture have nothing to do with the cause of this raised blood pressure. They just have two things for any kind of hypertension irrespective of its cause. And these two magical things are a standard advice which says not to take fried, salt & ghee, and a standard tablet. This difference in medical culture & medical science is the main culprit.

Note:

One thing I would like to clarify here; that doctors are neither foolish nor dumb. They are highly qualified and they represent most noble profession in this world. They have to study very hard from their school time just to crack and entrance exam, only then they could make the way clear for medical college. Things not end here; the academic decorum they have to pursue in their medical colleges is even designed to

polish their mental abilities. It is not fair to call them "idiots" either. Every child since his childhood at least once surely has a dream to become a doctor; this dream of becoming a doctor tells the dignity of this profession. Every pathy has gems and devils in it, so as with this allopathic system also. My emphasis is only that they are just ignorant, instead of working as per science they are actually working as per the system.

Chapter – 5
Idiopathic, Genetics & Idiots

Many common diseases today are believed for having unsure or unknown cause. In medical world very beautiful and relevant word is given to this, they call it idiopathic. Any disorder having unknown cause is known as an idiopathic disorder. Low back pain, diabetes, certain types of fever, sclerosis, some types of inflammation, renal disorders, mental disorder, epilepsy and many more disease are called idiopathic. Idiopathic actually means that the reason for occurrence of these diseases is unknown. Now this is amazing in simple words they are just saying that we don't know the cause of diseases but we have medicine to treat this disorder. This will heal your disease & that unknown cause will also be gone. They believe some chemical salts will fix everything and that unknown cause will also be corrected automatically. This is the biggest mistake our modern medical model is making and instead of being sorrow, they actually believe that their study & their work are very intelligent. In my opinion, the biggest threat to humans is this medical model because we are trusting on those professionals who actually don't know the exact cause of even fever. They are just trained to attack fever or mild pain associated with fever with their so called safest tablet known as paracetamol. In many countries, significant work & research have proved that paracetamol is deadliest form of medicine which is being used frequently in not only adults & children but in infants also. Modern doctors are believed to look at fever as a green headed monster which will kill or damages the body; but in fact, fever is a smart action or response of your body to fight with any kind of disease causing agent, by giving paracetamol we are hitting our body with double sided knife. By lowering body's temperature we are reducing body's own defense mechanism & on the other hand, we are hurting our body with paracetamol's side effects, which includes damage to the internal intestinal lining, liver, kidney etc. This also affects blood's defense chemistry by lowering production of extra W.B.C's which is body's Army to fight against diseases. Let me explain one of the biggest side effect of giving paracetamol in pain or other inflammatory disorders like arthritis, spondylitis, tendonitis, frozen shoulder etc. Paracetamol destroys ***'Glutathione'*** which is a strongest anti-oxidant of our body; no other medicine destroys 'Glutathione' like paracetamol. Glutathione is required to repair damaged cells of liver, it also helps in repairing cartilage of joints & connective tissues of skin, and it also reduces oxidative stress of the body. It also improves insulin resistance and pancreatic endocrine function. Glutathione is also a strong anti-oxidant to fight against various autoimmune disorders like rheumatoid arthritis, celiac disease as it protects and improves mitochondrial activity by reducing free radical load in body. You may be surprised that clogged artery & peripheral artery disease is also caused by deficiency of 'Glutathione'. If a pregnant lady is given paracetamol then it adversely affects the Nervous system of the child by increasing the levels of oxidative damage & lowering the level of 'Glutathione' in the brain. This is also a contributing factor for Autism in children. Reducing or destroying 'Glutathione' from the body may results in disordered metabolic activity & immune response, which may results in weak control over diabetes & respiratory disorders respectively. So, the bottom line is, "Paracetamol is very safe medicine as per modern doctors as it reduces fever & in return it destroys your liver cells, decreases immune response, weakens up cartilages of joints, reduces fever of mother for few hours & destroys brain cell of her child forever". It also damages digestion and absorption process of the body & interferes with the working of insulin. If you are taking paracetamol in joint pain, you are destroying your joint and its cartilages just to get a pain relief effect for maximum 8-10 hours. This is the reason why they call osteoarthritis an incurable disorder because the treatment they are having for knee joint pain is actually causing damage to the cartilage of the joint. This means, on the name of treating knee pain we are just suppressing the pain and damaging that joint in return. I must say modern science is not modern in any way.

Now coming next to the genetic cause of disease, I am sure many of you must be heard a word genetic cause in respect to many diseases like obesity, diabetes, hypertension or other life style disorders. This actually doesn't make any sense, in other words; they are saying you are fatty because your grandfather had eaten lots of sugar & fat in his lifetime. Grading a lifestyle disorder under genetic cause is very idiotic thing because you are demotivating a patient by saying him that you can't change this because it is not happened to you by your faulty eating habits or your sedentary lifestyle. You are fatty because of your grandfather. You have no way out to reverse this, all you can do is to take this medicine lifelong it will provide you a healthy and prosperous life; with time to time you will be advised to increase the dose of this medicine. Doesn't it sound silly & I am astonished that our society still believes on such kind of silly logics given by these health ambassadors. Before we directly jump on a conclusion that obesity or diabetes is caused by genetics always, just ask yourself can you really imagine a person who is following a low carbohydrate & low sugar diet format, running & exercising daily & does not have sedentary lifestyle but still having diabetes or obesity. You can never find a single person in your lifetime suffering from such diseases without faulty lifestyle or eating habits. Before tagging any disease as genetic, our modern doctors' needs to study "EPIGENETICS" which clearly says gene expression & carrying a gene are totally different cases. Gene expression depends upon nutrition, lifestyle, geographical area etc. In simple words, if someone is carrying a gene of any disease it will not be expressed unless you give a favorable outside environment for that disease to proliferate. It's just like a seed; underground waiting for its favorable condition outside, so that the seed could germinate and grows up as a plant or a tree. Always remember, "**Genetics load the gun but lifestyle puts the trigger**". On the whole, genetic cause & idiopathic factors are just two fancy terms used by your doctor to hide their ignorance or unawareness. Such words are expected to be used only by quacks or idiots but not by our highly qualified so called specialists & health professionals representing the most evolved, advanced & trusted system of healthcare.

Allopathic Genetic vs. Mendel's Genetics:

Sir Gregor Mendel, he was the father of genetics and gifted this world, the science of genetics by his incredible studies and experimentation in this particular field. Genetics is the science, which studies heredity and characteristics that are inherited from parents to the offspring. Mendel gave law of genetics which describes in detail how genetics works. He gave many laws regarding this particular field of biology. In context to today's allopathic doctor's genetic sense, I can say Mendel's genetics is totally against the theory of genetics being announced by them. Mendel's law says, any trait which is present in the parents will be transferred to the offspring in a progressive manner. In simple words, only superior characters will be transferred from a parent generation to their children. Any character which is faulty or disease causing will be diminished in next generation and eventually such characters will be vanished after few generation gaps. On the other hand, we are facing a burst of so called genetic disorders which were seen never before. Diabetes, obesity, arthritis, auto-immune disorders were not present 500 years ago, even before 100 years such disease were hardly witnessed. But from last few decades almost every so called genetic disorder is becoming epidemic. What kind of genetics is this? How a faulty character could starts expressing itself all of sudden and in an increasing order. Mendel will also be surprised, if he could see that how genetics has made a U-turn in modern world.

Coming straight to the point, genetics never works like this way.

Calcium Confusion:

This topic also deserves to be discussed as there is also very big misconception among not only layman but physicians also, that calcium makes bones healthier. Many companies are advertising their calcium supplements which are being sold at shining prices & believed to protect your bones and health as well, but it is not that simple. There are many factors which are responsible for bone health. You will be surprised to know that only 21 percent of our bones are contributed by Calcium. Rest of 80 percent is never talked about or I believes even most of the health professional are not even aware of this. More than 30 different minerals, proteins, connective tissues, lipids collectively make up a bone structure. This is silly that only calcium tablet is going to fix any kind of disorder related to bones. Another drawback in this theory is the kind of calcium you are being offered within those tablets. No matters how cheap or costly type of calcium tablets you are purchasing, those tablets contains calcium carbonate (CaCO3) which is a type of stone, and we know it as lime stone. This is very harmful type of calcium. Our body cannot metabolize calcium carbonate as it is not the type of calcium your body needs. Some companies are providing calcium citrate tablets; same story with these tablets also. On the other hand, you must know calcium is lethal killer in today's world from renal stones to fatal heart attacks; calcium is a main concerned culprit. There is a great book by "Dr. Thomas Levy, M.D." named "Death By Calcium", I highly recommend this book as this book offers scientific proof that how the regular intake of dairy & other calcium supplementation promotes all known chronic degenerative diseases & shortens life significantly. But look at our conventional medical doctors; they are still considering calcium as a superman's molecule which will shield bones and joints from any threat.

I am not even saying that calcium should not be used at all. My concerns are only to use calcium, if you are really deficient of it and never ever use that toxic calcium carbonate in attractive packing. Calcium from raw milk (not processed because processed milk is dangerous for our body), nuts, some vegetables, pulses or organic pasture-raised eggs are the best source of natural calcium. Iron

Iron Tablets (Ferrous Sulphate):

This is another toxic form of medicine being distributed freely by our modern doctors. The type of iron which they use in their tablets is like small molecule of iron bonded with sulphur and oxygen molecules. Which means it is the heaviest form of iron powdered up & shaped into a tablet or a capsule. Though, it increases little iron content in body but it also agitates immune response of our body; as body recognizes it as a foreign iron piece or a foreign body inside the system. That's why it is often noted that if we use these iron tablets in patients; colitis or other inflammation of gastro intestinal track (G.I.T.) symptoms aggravates very quickly and sometimes patient even develops bleeding with stool. If such iron tablets are taken regularly patient may develop some kind of auto-immune disorders as these tablets generates a massive immune response. Instead of prescribing such toxic form of iron, patient must be advised to take natural iron source from diet which includes raw milk, dark green leafy vegetables, beat root, pomegranate, avocado, nuts & many other natural veg & non-veg sources.

Idiopathic fever & Antibiotics:

Certain types of fever having unknown cause or what they say idiopathic fever is still a mystery for modern medical system. In fact, they are not educated well that why body gets fever. They are only trained to normalize fever & this is a job at which they are good enough. But they are not taught that fever is beneficial and sometimes it is body’s physiological need to have slightly raised temperature which needs not to be suppressed with medicines always. As season changes, body sometimes need extra W.B.C. to withstand this change & be prepared for upcoming season. Usually, this is done at normal body temperature but if our immunity is already struggling or body is deficient of any certain nutrient; body needs little rise in temperature to make this reaction fast. This kind of fever will not be traced in any lab investigation or blood reports and it will be named Idiopathic fever. From here onwards, a new story begins, once this fever is misrecognized as a disease or symptom, they will try their best to pull this fever down. They will use antibiotics, antipyretics & many such allopathic medicines to bring this fever down to normal. Now, let's calculate the damage to the body by this, First thing which will happen is, body will fail to produce that extra immune cells regarding which this temperature was being raised. On the other hand, antibiotics will affect adversely to the gut and gut-flora where 70 percent of your body's Immunity lives. Gut needs a huge colony of friendly bacteria for providing immunity to the body, but antibiotics are cutting immunity just to treat that fever superficially that was meant to improve immunity of the body. The natural fever has to be down by itself within 24-48 hours, but antibiotics will stretch this fever for months long. Antibiotics are not always dangerous but while practicing medicine 90 percent of our doctors misuse it in ignorance. I am not saying that they are knowingly misusing it but they are actually unaware about exact effect of antibiotics and its damaging effect to the body. In fact, some doctors even believe using a higher class of antibiotic will benefit the patient and helps him to heal rapidly.

Good & Bad NEWS Regarding Cancer:
Cancer is always a threat to humanity and a nightmare for medical industry. It is the only disease which is ranked at the top of all deadliest diseases known to the mankind. Ever since our medical industry is working on cancer, huge amount of money is flooded in the research regarding cancer treatment. Unfortunately, it is still second biggest cause for deaths in the United States. Since last 20 years, it is growing in developing countries like India also. After many researches what our medical field is considering as valid and authentic treatment for cancer is a chemotherapy or radiotherapy. Maybe you are aware of it or not that people are dying early and in a bigger number with this chemotherapy as compared to cancer itself. So, it means we have a treatment for cancer which helps us to die early. This is happening because we have not understood cancer cells yet.

Cancer is a disease like a silent terrorist attack on the body. We must understand this thing before taking any action against cancer. Now imagine a situation when a bunch of terrorists are inside your territory, what kind of actions should be taken to kill them? Would you prefer to use a bomb or go for sniper who can shoot bullet accurately on their head? Using a bomb will hurt your own people inside that territory more than the terrorists. We all know this will not work, but surprisingly we are using same chemical bombs and radio bombs to kill some cancerous cell inside our body and the results are also unexpected. Healthy cells of our body are also being affected badly with this chemotherapy treatment. We need to look for some kind of sniper method while treating cancer.

I am stupefied to think that how chemotherapy and radiotherapy is regarded as a valid treatment for treating cancer. It is very basic thing that cancer grows in body when immunity goes down. Strong immune cells will never allow cancerous cells to grow in our body. You have no right to do such stupidity on cancer patients because chemotherapy will totally destroy the immunity of the body. To headshot cancer cells, we just need to know cancer cells and its working. One thing which is sure about cancer cells is they need 20 times more glucose than the normal cells of the body. Another thing which we know is, it can survive only in an anaerobic medium. Cancer cells needs to divide very rapidly & this kind of fast metabolism could be only supported by an acidic medium only. Cancer cell requires heavy blood supply to proliferate, that's why extra channel of blood vessels is developed around cancer cells. In order to kill cancer cells we should design a strategy which can affect all the above mentioned factors supporting cancerous growth. What if I say that cancer is not untreatable, only we are treating it in a bad manner. We have designed a treatment which is helping patients to die in a legal way by spending huge amount of money just to insert some chemicals in the body which provides toxicity and a well decorated death in a big reputed hospital. Another benefit of such kind of poisonous treatment for cancer is; it gives a sense of satisfaction to the relatives and family members of the patient that they had tried their best. Other than this nothing good is happening with such kind of ridiculous treatment.

So let's move towards the good news regarding cancer, which I can call a sniper method. We all know we have to attack on basic points which support cancer.

`Acidic medium of body should be converted into basic medium.

`Glucose supply to the cancerous cells should be cut off.

`Immunity of the body should be promoted with all the known methods; only then we can attack cancerous cells.

Body should be supplied with enormous amounts of oxygen to hinder anaerobic mode of cancer cells.

Cancer treatment is actually complicated that if we go for detailed approach a whole independent book only on cancer could be devoted. But here I will give you just a bird's eye view or nutshell approach which will definitely improve your understanding regarding cancer.

Diet:

Diet should be consisting of at least 70 percent of alkaline food because as per "Warburg effect" cancer cells grow and divides more rapidly in an acidic & anaerobic medium. Diet should be extremely fresh with very low quantity of sugar in it. Fresh food contains high amount of anti-oxidants which helps body to promote immunity and reduces oxidative stress in body. Anything containing refined sugar, refined oil, refined salt, refined flour or any kind of processed food should be strictly eradicated from diet. Another thing which is extremely important regarding diet is when to eat. Remember what and when are two basic stands on which an ideal diet is placed. Eating window is the basic tool regarding when to eat, 24 hours of a day must be divided into two phases, first phase is eating phase & second phase is fasting phase. Normally eating phase should not exceed by one third of the fasting phase which means we should maintain eating window of 6 hours and rest of 18 hours must be a fasting phase. These 6 hours of eating should be any time from a 24 hours day. In my practice, I usually recommend patients to make this fasting window from 11:00 am to 4:00 pm. Shorter this eating window higher will be the success rates. I use 5 hours eating window with my patients, this window could be relaxed up to 8 hours & constricted up to 3 hours. Let's assume if a person starts eating at 6 or 7 AM in the morning and takes his last meal, snack, tea-coffee, cookies or anything at 10 or 11 pm, so this is a window of 17 to 18 hours which is more than a worst dietary habit. Though our modern society is filled with a rumor which is telling us to take small & divided meals throughout the day but this was never supported by any doctor or any Research Centre. Because eating in small quantities & repeatedly will result in dis-balanced physiology of body & keep you in a digestive phase always, which will ultimately slowdowns rejuvenation and repair process of the body, not only regarding cancer: this kind of diet is harmful for everyone.

Autophagy: Power of Fasting:

Almost everyone is familiar with fasting but most of them know little or nothing regarding this. Fasting: if done with proper guidance and method can give numerous benefits to our body. This is not a health tip or some kind of alternate therapy but it is a complete treatment in itself. It promotes repair process in body, helps in reducing weight, detox & remove toxics from body and liver also, it also helps in reducing insulin resistance and other markers of hyper-insulinemia, reduces chronic inflammation, improves brain function & helps to fight with other mental conditions like Alzheimer's. Not only this, it also boosts immunity & helps to stay young. Almost in every culture & every religion fasting is significantly advised, as while fasting body works on itself rather than doing digestion & other biochemical reaction needed to absorb and metabolize food.

To understand fasting more efficiently, I would like to give an example here. If you are busy in going to office daily without holiday, you would hardly manage other domestic things to be completed like preparing breakfast, kitchen management & other routine stuff. But, in this hectic schedule you may ignore your backyard or some other repair work in your home like painting or some other maintenance work. Because going office daily after completing other basic domestic work has booked you up completely. Similarly, digestion is very big process for your body and it uses up all the energy of body in digesting food, absorbing and utilizing it. Similarly, if you give your body a leave from its daily work; body will definitely repair itself. But we are not supporting our body to do so. We are continuously engaging our body in digesting something, not only this, before sleeping we put some more food or snacks or milk inside the stomach which means you are saying to your body that I am going for a sleep but you must work on this digestion process and everything should be digested before I awake. This is a rude manner and disrespect to this wonderful self-healing design what we call human body. Fasting must be done with water only, if we are taking juices or fruits during this fasting phase that is not what fasting is. Ideally, fasting could be done like the window system which is discussed earlier in this chapter. Other methods of fasting includes:-

1) Fasting on every alternate day.
2) Three days- only water fast in a week.
3) Five days- only water fast continuously, once in a month.

Insulin, Obesity & Insulin Resistance:

Obesity and diabetes are two biggest undefeated dragons in our today's world. Though many inventions and latest medicines have been invented to control these two disorders but nothing looks like working. Obesity & diabetes are fundamentally misunderstood. We are only looking at our diet but ignoring a biggest phenomenon behind this, which is hormonal alignment. Anything we eat behaves in our body as per our hormones & bio-chemistry. I am sure, if we can understand these two diseases up to the level of hormones, fear of diabetes & failure in weight loss will be vanished away. I will move step by step to explain where we are missing basic concepts regarding these two diseases; till the end of the topic you will definitely get a detailed approach over it.

Insulin:

Insulin is a hormone which is secreted by pancreas in response to glucose or carbohydrate in our body. Main function of insulin is to metabolize glucose in our blood. Insulin is a key hormone which allows sugar to enter into the cell. In the absence of insulin, blood glucose cannot enter into the cell. This is the condition which could be called type II diabetes. Insulin spikes up when your meal contains heavy sugar or carbohydrates in it. Every time you eat something the insulin level goes up. Insulin spike tells the body to store energy within the cells, more the insulin spikes; higher the tendency of body to store energy. So, obesity is directly related with insulin or we can say insulin spike. Obesity has nothing to do with calorie counting which will be discussed further in detail. Insulin spike depends on Glycemic Index (GI) of food. Every foodstuff has a certain glucose producing capacity which is measured on a scale called Glycemic Index. Fats & Proteins are very low at glycemic Index whereas carbohydrates like potato, wheat, corn and other cereals are very high in Glycemic Index. If we talk about refined sugar, beverages, white flour or other kind of processed food, insulin spike will go over the roofs. If your body is high on insulin you are definitely going to store energy and will gain weight eventually. On the other hand, if you have lower insulin levels in body you will face a hard time to gain weight. Anything which touches insulin level in your body can affects your body's weight directly. Let's look at an example for better understanding over this topic: We know steroids have a side effect of weight gain. So does weight gain with steroid is happening without Insulin? Steroids like prednisolone put a paddle on sympathetic nervous system of the body which tells body to break down more glycogen and produce glucose. Which is understood as steroids raises blood glucose level, that's why steroids are primary treatment of hypoglycemic conditions. This glucose rise with steroid generates a strong insulin spike & we gain weight as a result. Same story could be implemented if a person is high on cortisol hormone (stress hormone) because cortisol is the natural corticosteroid of the body. This is the reason we must check stress levels of patient while treating diabetes & obesity. Because this cortisol will spike blood glucose level & Insulin levels in the body.

Obesity:

Before starting obesity, let us look at the traditional way of calorie counting method again. Calorie is the unit of fuel inside our body; fuel brunt is directly proportional to the energy produced is a law of physics. We call it "Law of Thermodynamics". But, this law doesn't works inside human body because there is a whole new mechanism; we call it metabolism or biochemistry. Look again, what this calorie counting method is saying. According to this, if we are eating a plate of salad or a plate of pasta or sugar loaded food like ice-cream or candies and all of them are exactly same in calorific value. Your body will behave exactly same in the terms of energy production. This is the most stupid theory regarding human body. If we take olive oil & pastries equal in calories both will behave same inside the body & produces equal amount of energy this is what this theory states. This is the reason, people struggle lifetime with obesity and spend half of their precious time in calculating calories. God knows! who did this useless work and created such a mess by raising this defected theory. Weight loss could be done easily if you are able to lower insulin levels in body.

Another lie regarding weight loss is some dieticians are spreading this fake information that eating in small intervals and divided meals is healthy. Again, same science while having small meals, insulin is secreted and snaking or small divided meals will promote insulin release again & again. When I hear to any so called health expert advising to take small meals again & again 8 to 10 times a day, I feel pity for their patients. Such diet experts have no clue how human body works. Methods to cut insulin level from body are based on two basic pillars; first is what to eat & second is when to eat. Just take only one or two standard basic meals, no snacking should be done in between and the diet must be extremely low in carbohydrates & sugars.

Let's be logical on Genetic Disorders:

Before 1900 no-one was talking about genetic disorder. In fact, obesity & diabetes originated in last 50-70 years. So, what kind of genetic is this, which was not present in our ancestors but it is developing in their off springs? This sense of genetics is completely against the “Law of Genetics" given by G. Mendel (Father of Genetics) & Darwin (Theory of Evolution). Darwin Theory of evolution states that faulty gene or inferior factors will be vanished or diminished in next off springs. Which means these genetic disorders should be higher in previous generations & must be reduced in next generations, but the case here is totally opposite. Allopathic doctors are saying that these genetic disorders are getting worsen & increasing in numbers generation after generations. Let me inform you one thing more, they never cross checked their doubt for genetic cause of such diseases they just assume & believe their assumptions. If these diseases are really genetic, then can they explain that before 100 years where these diseased genes were locked? This whole theory of genetic is result of their negligence.

Let me explain what is happening here. Have you seen a printer which prints different colors on a paper exactly same as a master copy but if this printing machine is deficient of any one colored ink, it will still print but this time, printed copy will be altered in colors from master copy. This is the same case happening with their so called genetic disorders. When we are deficient in certain minerals, vitamins or other nutrients, our gene still expresses themselves; but our body is out of certain nutrients required to this gene. Now, it will express itself in a faulty way. This is known as mutation in scientific language but our modern medicine puts everything on your side just to hide their failures.

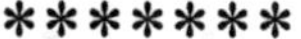

Chapter – 6
Missed topics in Modern Medicinal Curriculum

Modern medicine system being such a developed & research base science had undergone a very long journey. In this journey, many significant inventions are made which had served the humanity but still this medicine system has failed to heal our sick society. In fact, in other words, it could be said that many minor health issues when treated with modern medicine turn into a lifelong chronic disease. This is because there are some important sections which are ignored badly in their studying & learning process. We will discuss each of them one by one in this chapter.

Building up Immunity:

Though modern medicine admits that everything in the body depends upon immunity; from wound healing to fighting up with cancer or from any allergic disorder to communicable diseases, it's all dependent on how well our immune system is working. But till date, they are unaware of what kind of food actually boosts immunity directly. Neither boosting immunity is included in their study nor has even a single medicine been developed to increase immunity of the body. They are just trained to kill bacteria with antibiotics, kill inflammation with anti-inflammatory drugs or steroids but boosting immunity is still not under their command. Many researchers are now proving in their researches that nutrients like Vitamin C, Zinc, Selenium, Glutathione are strongest immune boosters but use of such nutrients are still not popular in modern healthcare system. I would like to share one more amazing facts concerning Vitamin C & immunity. As per medical text books, daily required dose of Vitamin C is between 1000-1500 mg and this dose was decided only in context of scurvy disease. This dosage is not sufficient when we are talking about anti-oxidant effect of Vitamin C. Normal dose while treating immune disorders should be between 10,000-30,000 mg orally. A modern medicinal doctor may snatch his head after imagining this dose in tablet form. But, there were many doctors in history, who have successfully treated patients with immune disorders even like "AIDS" by administrating high doses of Vitamin C. We must know that every animal except 'Human beings' and 'Guinea pig' produces Vitamin C inside the body to fight with diseases e.g. A goat produces more than 60,000 mg of Vitamin C daily in her body. Only human beings have to take it externally but this information is not delivered to us.

Note:

Chemical which is being sold on the name of Vitamin C is not actually Vitamin C; this is Ascorbic Acid or Sodium Ascorbate. Both of them have different molecular formula; they are not identical to naturally occurring Vitamin C which has a unique pattern of its molecule and also behaves very differently. Naturally occurring Vitamin C is L-Ascorbate or Ascorbium and its best sources are Indian Gooseberry fruit (Amla), lime, tamarind, guava, green chilies, goat milk, pineapple, kiwi fruit.

Healing up the System V/s Medicating a symptom:

This is another major fundamental mistake being made by our modern medical system that they ignored the importance of rejuvenation very badly. They are not taught how a system or an organ could be healed rapidly. This entire medical model is designed to drug the symptoms. Such kind of practice is hurting health of our society. What is happening under this system is they give medicine for one disease & disturbs working of many systems. Let's assume a person is being medicated for allergic disorders with anti-histaminic or anti-allergic drugs. Such drugs will temporarily reduce allergic reactions resulting in many side effects minor & major. Minor side effects are those which could be witnessed after few hours of consuming such medicines which includes dry mouth, dizziness, drowsiness, nervousness & mental irritability but if someone is consuming such medicines for regular & long period; symptoms could be very severe. Anti-allergic drugs affect adversely on sympathetic nervous system, adrenal glands & allergic response of our body. This could make allergy more severe by suppressing immune response. Endocrine system will be affected resulting various kind of hormone dis-balance; thyroid function & insulin responses will be altered

& list could be more long also. All this is happening because we have decided to fight allergy with anti-histamines rather than boosting immunity as allergy is a result of weak immune system. This was just an example, as every medicine used in allopathic system has same story: Anti-cholesterol medicines weakens the heart & is also a leading cause of arteriosclerosis & atherosclerosis, anti-depressant medicines cause severe depression & suicidal tendency, long term effect of multivitamins is lethargy & general weakness & so on. Let's assume if a patient is having liver or kidney disorders they have not developed any single effective medicine which could repair liver cells or nephrons of kidney. That's why a bigger section of our society is on dialysis & other severe liver disorders.

This system of drugging the symptoms is like fighting with a knife without safety handle. No doubt this knife may hurt the enemy but your hand will also be injured more.

Lack of Wholistic Approach:

Another rudimentary mistake our modern medical model had made is they are having specializations in different categories. Our body is actually one major system which is driven by collective actions of many sub systems. Each system is directly connected with the working of another system & is affected directly. Disorder of one system will produce direct symptom in other system because it is compensatory action of body or in medical term we call it homeostasis. But when we are trained to look at only one system without knowing its relation with other systems; mistakes could be guaranteed. Only one disordered system can alters the working of many other systems at same time. For making my point firmer; let's discuss an example: A patient is eating processed and junk food which will cause inflammation in the gut. This inflamed gut will cause hyperactivity in adrenal glands to produce cortisol (cortisol is strongest anti-inflammatory agent produced in body). Raised cortisol levels will activate sympathetic nervous system & make some changes, which will be increased blood pressure, reduced thyroid function, reduced digestion, increased cholesterol levels, elevated blood glucose levels, insomnia & anxiety. Now guess what, how a medical doctor will treat this patient. Endocrinologist will recommend him thyroxin tablet as TSH & T3, T4 will be found low. This doctor has no idea that thyroid works like see-saw with adrenals. This is how our body works if adrenals go up, thyroid function has to fall down & if thyroid is over active our adrenals have to sit down calmly. After endocrinologist, cardiologist will come & contributes his knowledge by recommending anti-cholesterol medications. He will also suggest that patient to take blood thinner and anti-hypertensive medicine regularly to secure his heart. Also, he will advise to take medicine for diabetes as his blood glucose is also raised. Rather than restricting inflammatory food and treating only gut inflammation, our modern medical system will mess this case so badly & the patient will be advised to take anti-cholesterol medicine, blood thinner, anti-hypertensive and a thyroid tablet regularly. Let me admit one thing very clearly here I am not against allopathic system or any healthcare system. I am only against stupidity and Idiotic actions.

Sympathetic Dominance State (Fight or Flight Mode):

Sympathetic Dominance state is body's normal response towards stress. There are mainly three types of stress: Physical, Chemical & Emotional. Body cannot differentiate between these three types of stress. Any kind of stress among these three activates sympathetic system of the body in which body alters its normal physiological process in a certain way.

Physical stress includes any kind of physical injury in present or past like accident or surgery. Chemical stress is the stress cause by toxics in the body which may come from adulteration in food, use of insecticide & pesticide, impure water, regular use of chlorinated water, allopathic medicines, toxic metal in food or drinking water, refined sugar, use of spray perfumes & uncountable, unwanted chemicals that we are encountering daily. Refined oils & processed cheese are also big cause of chemical stress. Third type of stress is emotional stress which is a result of emotional injury like bad social reputation, domestic violence, loss of loved one etc.

When your body is under any kind of stress, certain systems of the body directly gets concerned. This state is also called "fight or flight state". Let's understand this situation with a perfect example. If a person in a jungle is being chased by a tiger for the survival of the body. Fight or Flight mode will be activated to increase the chances of survival. Body will try to ensure all physical needs for escape from this situation. Blood sugar of body will be increased to supply continuous sufficient energy for running; cholesterols will also be raised, as while running, any cut or bleed may happen. This cholesterol will block and repair ruptured tissues or artery, respiration rate will also be increased to ensure sufficient oxygen in blood to generate enormous amount of extra energy required for the running. All these changes will be made by raised cortisol level, that's why in stress; cholesterols, blood sugar and sometimes respiration rate will go higher. On the other hand, digestive system, appetite & excretion will be delayed because if the tiger is chasing a person running away will be the priority of body and body will not choose rest & digest mode at that time. That's why hypothyroidism, weak digestions or loss of appetite, I.B.S. or constipation are also some side-effects of stressful state. Only fixing stress cause will improve all the symptoms in the body simultaneously.

Now let's calculate what does it means to be in a stressful state. You may have symptoms like high blood pressure, high blood glucose, raised cholesterol level, hypo functional thyroid & muscular pains but your doctor will give you a colorful pill for every symptom except pointing out the root cause, which is stress. Now guess, what effect will all those medications can have on your stress levels? Most of you may guess that stress level will remain the same or untouched which is also not a wrong statement but the most dangerous thing is with all these medications you are putting the body in more stressful condition because as described earlier these medications act as chemical triggers for stress. Are you getting me: What does it means? We are creating diseases in our society with such kind of healthcare system which is actually designed to keep hospitals full.

Another aspect of sympathetic dominance state or stressed condition is body produces heavy amounts of acid especially lactic acid & uric acid. When body is under adrenal dominant state symptoms related to excess acid will also be visible. These symptoms may include premature graying of hair, skin allergies, rashes etc. Now look at your surroundings, how many people are actually under stressful state and taking medicines for gout, arthritis, thyroid, high blood pressure, diabetes, skin allergies because of misdiagnosis of his medical doctor. Tablets of thyroid, diabetes, hypertension etc. are being distributed by these ignorant doctors like a sweet candy.

I dream of a society where, if a patient visits to doctor with raised cholesterol levels and high blood pressure. His doctor explains him to avoid all inflammatory foods from diet & tells him that he is under chemical stress state, in response to this stress his body has raised blood sugar to meet extra energy need and cholesterol levels are raised because body needs more cortisol to fight with inflammation. In order to produce cortisol, your body needs cholesterol as raw material. You just need to stick on healthy diet and proper sleep. Our society really needs such doctors, who can benefit the society and not the hospitals. Hoping for the best!

Nutrition and Detox:

At a cursory glance, it seems our modern science emphasis very well on the nutritional side of health but if we dig into it, this could be easily seen that nutritional side of health is significantly ignored. Modern science never looks at role of fortified nutrients in chronic disorders and always tries to suppress only the symptoms with allopathic medicine. Most of the diseases; nowadays is a kind of deficiency. We can see in the last 40 years, diseases and health statics is getting worsens day by day. There was a scientist in early 90's who states that there is no disease in humans which could not be related with some kind of deficiency in the body. Which means any disease could be healed only with fulfilling the deficient nutrient. In last 40 years, our soils are getting poor in minerals day by day. We call our soil motherland because of very strong reasons, soil is the only source from where all nutrients goes into our vegetables, fruits, cereals, animal products or anything you can imagine as your food. But if soils are getting bad in nutrients human sufferings will be significantly increased. This is what we are seeing in last 3-4 decades. Most of the fertile lands are now loaded with chemicals such as fertilizers, insecticides, pesticides etc. So in such a dark age of healthcare; nutritional side of diseases must be researched and cured. We must know that if we give our body all the required nutrients, body can handle its issues well. Never forget your body is designed to heal by itself and to live on this planet. All you have to do is feed your body with each & every nutrient which is more than toughest job in such time when we are consuming genetically modified foods, taking allopathic medicines regularly, our soils are running out of nutrients regularly, our diary and other animal products are loaded with artificial hormones, we are dependent on artificially ripened fruits & this list is not stopping.

Our nutrition is divided into 5 major sections which are: -

1) Glucose
2) Vitamins
3) Minerals
4) Proteins & Amino Acids
5) Fats or Fatty Acids.

This could be further classified into two main sections.

1) Essential Nutrients
2) Non-Essential Nutrients

Essential Nutrients:

Essential nutrients are those which are not synthesized in the body and you have no other choice except taking it orally. These nutrients could not be produced in body and we are bound to take it in our food or in the form of some herbal, non-fortified and natural supplements.

Non-Essential Nutrients:

Non-essential nutrients are those which could be synthesized in the body so we don't have to worry much about them.

Let's talk about essential nutrients in detail, as we have to include them in our daily menu.

Essential Nutrients:

There are total 90 nutrients which are essential for our body neither less nor more. If we are able to fetch all these 90 nutrients in right amount no health issue could run for a long period of time in body. 'Dr. Wallach' who is a naturopathic doctor from U.S.A. had done marvelous work in this direction. He explained all the essential & non-essential nutrients in very detailed and practical way.

Glucose or sugar is not essential to the body as our body can produce required amount at glucose by breaking proteins or fat. Many doctors are unaware of this thing & try to heal every disorder with glucose infusions, fruits, fruit juices or even simple glucose water; they prescribe such things to be taken orally. Fruits & fruit juices though I personally don't recommend but could be considered healthy, as it also contains some minerals & vitamins but giving glucose powder is not an intelligent approach. This is the reason that there are essential minerals, essential fatty acids, essential amino acids & essential vitamins but there is nothing like essential glucose or essential carbohydrate. Because our body can produce it and this process is called "Gluconeogenesis".

Note:
Gluconeogenesis is different from glycogenesis. Glycogenesis is production of glucose from glycogen whereas gluconeogenesis is when glucose is produced from proteins or fats.

There are total 90 essential minerals to be taken daily let's look at them.

60 Essential minerals:
Calcium, Magnesium, Phosphorus, Potassium, Sodium, Chlorine, Sulphur, Cobalt, Copper, Arsenic, Barium, Beryllium, Boron, Bromine, Carbon, Iodine, Iron, Manganese, Selenium, Zinc, Cerium, Cesium, Chrome, Dysprosium, Erbium, Europium, Gadolinium, Gallium, Germanium, Gold, Hafnium, Holmium, Hydrogen, Lanthanum, Lithium, Lutetium, Lead, Molybdenum, Neodymium, Nickel, Niobium, Nitrogen, Oxygen, Praseodymium, Rhenium, Rubidium, Samarium, Scandium, Silica, Silver, Strontium, Tantalum, Terbium, Thulium, Tin, Titanium, Vanadium, Ytterbium, Yttrium, Zirconium.

16 Essential Vitamins:
Vitamin A, Thiamine (B1), Riboflavin (B2), Niacin (B3), Pantothenic Acid (B5), Pyridoxine (B6), Cobalamin (B12), Vitamin C, Vitamin D, Vitamin E, Biotin, Choline, Flavonoids, Bioflavonoids, Folic Acid, Inositol.

12 Essential Amino Acids:
Lysine, Leucine, Valine, Threonine, Isoleucine, Tryptophan, Phenylalanine, Methionine, Histidine, Arginine, Taurine, Tyrosine.

2 Essential Fatty Acids:
Saturated & Unsaturated

Among all of the above; most difficult part nowadays, is to have those 60 minerals on daily basis in our diet. Though 16 vitamins, 12 Amino Acids & both fatty acids are also crucial to be added in our diet plan but somehow they could be attained by balancing and planning of diet. But biggest challenge is minerals because our body does not utilize artificially derived minerals properly. Plant based minerals has maximum bio-availability & our body absorbs and metabolizes it efficiently. Many Ayurvedic medicines can offer you most of these minerals and being plants based medicine, bio-availability and absorption will also be excellent. This is the reason where allopathic medicines produce side-effects and Ayurvedic medicine produces side-benefits; if it is prescribed by a qualified and expect Ayurvedic physician.

On the other hand, if we treat any deficiency symptom with allopathic medicines body will start losing its mineral reservoir more quickly because allopathic medicines are chemicals & our body needs extra army of nutrients to deal with those chemical based medicines. For example: increased heart rate could be balanced by just giving natural source of calcium (not calcium carbonate tablet). But, when we will try to balance it with some allopathic medicine like propanol or beta blockers, body will be affected adversely and may lead to some bigger cardiac issue in future.

Similarly, allergies and infections should be treated by increasing anti-oxidants and boosting immunity of the body, which could be done by giving high dose of Vitamin C, zinc, copper, selenium, sulphur in diet or medicinal form but choosing anti-allergic or anti-biotic & taking it for long period will agitate many vital biological processes of body resulting in weak immunity and you have chance to get those infections and allergies again & again.

Detox:

Modern science has never worked on detoxification of the system. There is no single medicine or any procedure which could contributes for detoxification of the body as explained earlier most of the diseases & disorders are due to toxics in our environment and body. Toxics are entering our system through drinking water, fruits & vegetables, processed foods etc. In our modern world, everything is contributing to make us sick & diseased. Detoxification gives our body a new start and improves rejuvenation inside our body. Let me explain, detoxification is not that easy as you might have heard, to just put some kind of stuff like lemon, mint, cucumber etc. in a jug full of water & drink it next morning. This could be beneficial in other ways as this water will carry many extra nutrients from the added stuff but it is given a name which doesn't goes well with its effect on body. There is nothing such miraculous component in it, which could be considered as an effective detoxifier. This is just mineralized water but calling it detox water is inappropriate.

To understand the science of detoxification, we must know that our body has appointed five organs which have the responsibility to detoxify our system.

Those five detoxifying organs are:-

1. Liver
2. Kidney
3. Skin
4. Lungs
5. Colon (Large Intestine)

Mild type of detoxifiers are those which influences at least two out of five above maintained detoxifying organs, Vitamin C & Rock salt is considered as a mild detoxifier as it slightly activates kidneys & colon resulting increased urine output and proper evacuation. But major part of detoxification is done by your liver and most importantly through skin. Your skin continuously throws out toxic chemicals through millions & millions of small pores in the skin. These toxic elements are seen on your clothes even in dust free environment, collars of shirt will turns shady. This is the waste of your body, which is thrown out from the skin. Now imagine, how many chemicals you are injecting into your body when you apply sun-screens or any other ointments on your skin. Anything you apply on your skin gets absorbed into the body or you can say your skin eats it up. This is the reason why Ayurveda never advices to put anything on your skin which could not be eaten.

Gall Bladder is useless, let's remove it:

This topic really astonishes me that how a bunch of doctors can decide and challenge the design of the creator. They believe removing gall bladder, in case of gall bladder stones is safe, how they can even ignore such a useful & important body part. Gall bladder is a store house of bile salts. When fat molecule strikes the stomach our gall bladder pushes out instantly required amount of bile into digestive system and this bile plays very important role in the breakdown of fat molecules. Breakdown of fat is very necessary for production of many hormones, essential fatty acid for nourishing the brain and different body parts. It is also required for the production of cortisol which is strongest form of steroid; our body requires fighting against inflammation and auto-immune disorders.

Let's calculate the effect of gall bladder removal now. Unfortunately, many doctors explain that having a removed gall bladder is usually safe. But, sometimes patients may complaint for some indigestion or minor gastric issues which is not true. Gall Bladder removal surgery can leads to many dangerous disorders like unhealed inflammation because body is now incapable of producing cortisol. You may witness many patients who have developed joint pains, muscular pains and other disorders after few years of gall bladder removal surgery. Now moving further, this may shock you but gall bladder removal in females is a significant cause of hormone dis-balance, estrogen dominance, uterine fibroids & even cancer. All these issues are caused because when body is high in estrogens and low on progesterone. Progesterone is produced from pregnenolone and pregnenolone is produced from cholesterols but we had blocked the production of cholesterols by removing gall bladder & fats are now not metabolized in the system efficiently. It means, hospital industry which is removing gall bladder today is compelling you to visit again for either a knee replacement surgery, uterus removal surgery or for a chemotherapy and radiotherapy. Does it make sense to you? After studying 8-10 years about human body and its diseases how they can mess this system so badly. They call it most advanced science because of latest surgical techniques that has been developed and I also agree on this. But, a simple gall bladder stone makes them so helpless that they found no way except cutting that gall bladder and throwing it out which is causing number of diseases afterwards. I hope no one would like to get a cancer just to prevent reoccurrence of gall bladder stones. I request all the mentors in the medical and surgery department to teach their trainee doctors that how important this gall bladder is. If it is really required to remove stones from gall bladder, I trust more than 100 percent on this modern healthcare system that they can definitely develop a surgery which will remove stones from gall bladder without removing gall bladder itself.

Doctors must look into it again, if they can remove the stones from gall bladder by just making an incision and removing out stones. Surgery is not my department, so I cannot suggest the technique. But being a physician, I just know that gall bladder is not an empty wrapper which is useless to body. We must know that, “In nature we cannot just do only one thing”. This will never go the way you perceive or the way you expect. In nature, everything is interconnected so as with the human body also. So, you really cannot make only one change. Let's understand it:

If it is nature or human body, no one can change just one thing because changing one thing will start a series of reaction which will change the system in number of ways. Let's imagine, if someone tries to stop any river or water channel towards any particular area. Is it possible that anything except that one river is not changed? No, it is not going to happen like this way. We can just stop a river but nature will make numerous adjustments just in response to this single change. Life around that river, fertility of surrounding land, type of plantation, speed of air, humidity of that area and almost everything will be affected. We just changed one thing but rest of the phenomenon is out of our control. Similarly, can you kill any one type of creature from this planet totally? Let's say rats; what will happen if all the rats got vanished all of sudden from this planet 'Earth'. You will observe a series of adjustments in nature from this single change. Many insects will start growing in population within few years, because these insects were supposed to be eaten up by those rats. This increase in the population of insects will further influence other creatures in number of ways and this reaction will keep expanding with time. Imagine any kind of example and the consequences will be found same every time. I am again reminding; you cannot change just one thing in nature.

In modern medicine, this important reality needs to be reminded because they believe with their chemical tablets they are just changing one thing. They believe that ant-acid tablets affect only acid of stomach and nothing else is changed in the body. By anti-hypertensive medicines, they are just lowering blood pressure of the body and again nothing else is affected. Diuretic tablets are just increasing quantity of urine and again nothing else is influenced. I have to say you are completely on a wrong track which will finally meet a dead end.

Chapter – 7
Why I Prefer Ayurvedic Perspective in Healthcare

In today's fastest growing healthcare when we are discovering more & more advanced medicines for different types of disorders. Advanced and higher generations of antibiotics are being discovered, treatment for diabetes or cardiovascular disorders are being updated continuously but, still it seems like something fundamentally went wrong with our inventions or discoveries. This is very astonishing thing that we are the generation who have highly advanced healthcare system & huge amount of health issues & untreatable diseases at the same time. If you look at it with a rational vision you will notice that the treatment or medicine, we are being advertised today as latest & effective medicine with least side effects. Only within 3-5 years surprisingly, these medicines will be tagged as outdated & dangerous medicines. I just mean, people are being used as laboratory mice; and they are being experimented for newer & newer medicines with fancy names just to see the effect of such toxic inventions by our healthcare system. The doctor who is prescribing you any medicine as latest and safer medicine will change his statement within 3-5 years only. Actually, this is the durability and reliability of allopathic medicines. Most of the medicines which were used by our healthcare system and doctors before 10 years are either ineffective or banned today & this is a fact.

On the other hand, Ayurvedic text was written almost 5000 years ago and still explains human health & diseases very accurately. Not even single word is outdated or incorrect till date. When you buy any electronic gadget the manufacturer company provides you a user manual which explains that gadget & its expected issues in an authentic way. Similarly, Ayurveda is that manual book from the creator for wellbeing of human race. In such a critical time, when our antibiotics are getting resistant, our painkillers are becoming ineffective, anti-fungal medicines are going in vain. Our human race strictly needs Ayurveda to be promoted as healthcare system. By looking at the current situation of allopathic system it could be clearly anticipated that this healthcare system is definitely going to collapse in next 15-20 years. Screwing up aluminum joints in knees & hips, implanting useless rings called stents inside blood vessels of heart or putting a major section of our society on chemical tablets; it is not an advanced science in any sense. It you start calling your bicycle as a sports car, it will make no difference with your bicycle's speed, performance or in anything. Similarly, calling such a damaging healthcare system as advanced science or modern science is doing nothing good for humanity.

Ayurveda states before creating human race god created medicines in the form of herbs & natural minerals. In support of this, there is also a very beautiful example to understand the importance of relation between herbal medicines and humans. I am translating you exact meaning of that example which says, "As a pregnant mother gets milk in her breast before her child come into existence, it is the same way god created herbs for nourishing and treating human beings." This is not an imaginary statement because our evolutionary science also tells us that plant kingdom arises first on this planet than animal kingdom. Unfortunately, many people assume that Ayurveda is a book for some kind of domestic cures & is not scientific; which is completely wrong.

Ayurvedic medicines are as safe as your food. Our body also recognizes and utilizes everything in its natural and non-synthetic form. Ayurveda is not what most of people thinks about it, like something mixed in honey or ghee could be beneficial in certain diseases. As per actual Ayurvedic text, every disease is divided into four basic parts which are based on its prognosis. First part is "Asadhya" which means untreatable, second one is "Krish-sadhya" which means it could be treated but with difficulty as it will need proper care & time to heal. Third category is "Yapya" which is the category in which; though we cannot heal the disease permanently but at least we can improve the symptoms with regular medicine & last one is "Susadhya" which means easily treatable. It is not like drinking a cup of green tea with all your same habits will lose some unimaginable pounds of weight within seven days or 10 days. Even types of cancer, medicines to cure, and prognosis of different type of cancer is also explained very well. The facts which is being discovered today after conducting million-dollar research is written in Ayurvedic texts 5000 years ago. Even diabetes, which is known to modern science in last 100 years, Ayurveda explains pre-diabetic symptom, diabetes & its expected complications along with proper treatment in that ancient time, which is really surprising. This is really beyond imagination; five thousand years ago, when most of the civilization over the world were eating raw leaves or such kind of stuff, many civilizations were not even able to invent clothes & used to cover themselves with some kind of leaves. At that time, Ayurveda was being documented as a written text in India. Most of the civilizations were not aware how to extract oil from seeds; Ayurveda was explaining different types of oils and qualities of each one of them. Nothing went wrong from that text till today. Whether it comes at symptoms or diseases treatment, eating habits, sleep patterns & almost everything is true and being proved right till date. Most of us may think logics and concepts are weaker sections in Ayurvedic science. 70 percent of Ayurvedic doctors chooses formula based practice, which means they directly chooses an Ayurvedic medicine for any health issue by completely ignoring body type, chronicity of diseases, types of symptoms and many other diagnostics steps which are important before jumping on to medicine selection.

Delinquency of Ayurvedic Doctors:

I feel ashamed for such Ayurvedic practitioners who are trying to practice Ayurveda in a mimicking style of allopathic system. Rudimentary point which I want to raise here is both sciences are completely different from each other and has their respective ethics of practice, selection of medicine; just looking at any symptom or disease is the way, how allopathic system works but this approach should not be used while practicing Ayurveda. Ayurveda is a personalized science which needs proper learning process, diagnostic skills & presence of mind. But mostly, we can see that Ayurveda is presented as some kind of relaxing spa therapies in which they proudly present themselves as a knowledgeable Ayurvedic doctors or Vaidyas by doing some kind of therapies. I am not against what they chooses to pursue as their profession but if they are doing some kind of therapies; then they must call themselves as an Ayurvedic therapist, rather than some kind of specialist or expert of Ayurvedic field because world will know Ayurveda only in the way this pathy is being carried by their successors.

India is a country who possesses the honor of representing Ayurveda in this whole world. But let's look at the ground report what is happening here actually. Every year thousands of students complete their Ayurvedic degree from various affiliated Institutions. After studying 5-6 years in the field more than 90 percent of them pass out with almost zero interest, faith & knowledge of Ayurveda. I am saying this with lots of grief & pain dipped heart that these doctors are very unaware of what does it really means to represent such a complete healthcare science. They are choosing to work as caretaker doctors in hospitals, where they are just hired to keep things in order and make sure that hospital staff is working properly. To my surprise, for such work they feel very proud of themselves. If someone is working in a heart care hospital, he declares himself as a cardiologist by his own. Similarly, after passing Ayurvedic degree we have bunch of so called cardiologists, nephrologists, neurologists among themselves. But, no one among them could be a complete Ayurvedic doctor. This is the biggest tragedy what Ayurveda is facing. As I said, this pathy belongs to creator himself this is the reason with all drawbacks in our educational system, this pathy is creating gems since ages and one in thousands of such gems are still being created till date. I bow myself completely to such "Master Healer Vaidyas" who are really born to serve humanity. If somehow, we can improve this section in which Ayurveda is being taught; I mean after completing education, if at least 50 percent of doctors can represent and practice Ayurveda in its original form. Nation will witness a golden era in healthcare. We can directly control this raising graph of lifestyle disorders and premature sudden deaths. Not only national diseases & health rate will be improved but also a very big amount of money could be saved within the country.

Western countries and other developed countries are promoting Ayurveda and significant improvements are also being visible now in various health sections. But doctors in India are stenting our society without hesitation and without actual needs. Our doctors hesitate to go for those procedures which are not profitable to the hospital, which includes normal delivery, avoiding unnecessary stents etc. This is the perfect time to invest on Ayurveda now.

Basic difference between allopathic and Ayurveda is; Allopathic system talks about suppress, kill pathogen, suppress that function, block some kind of receptors whereas Ayurveda talk about balance of 'Tridosh' and five basic elements which are present in body and universe as well.

Allopathic system is designed to get rid from diseases only; Ayurveda talks about preservation of health in healthy person, and curing the sick. So, everyone can live his life in a harmony with nature and meets to the ultimate destiny finally.

Commendable Sections in Modern Medicine: Everything has its both darker and brighter sides, so as with modern medicine also. There are many sections where modern medicine really deserves to be praised. In case of emergency conditions, allopathic system is really unmatchable. Many health conditions related with chronic infections like septicemia or other life threating infectious diseases, there is no such healthcare system which could be compared with the effectiveness of allopathic medicinal system. Though surgery is originally native to Ayurveda as it was discovered & practiced by an ancient Ayurvedic physician & surgeon called "Sushruta" but the way this surgery department is refined and evolved in allopathic system is really admirable. Latest surgical techniques, surgical equipment, aseptic environment & pre-post-operative care is really something this allopathic system should be applauded for. Another biggest achievement in modern science is development of advanced life care support & lifesaving medicines. Invention of anesthesia is a very big and worth achievement which adds feather in the hat of this modern medicine. If we talk about lifestyle disorders, Ayurveda has no comparison with any healthcare system in this world. It is most ancient and authentic science of life, similarly in emergency conditions allopathic system is really a boon. If both sciences work in their respective sectors our human race will again get rid from its suffering & health will start blossoming again. Both sciences need to recognize their stronger sides and focus on that also rather than indulging in unhealthy discussion and debates. Both sciences should work in the serving of human race rather than competing with each other. It is not like modern science belongs to those who are educated with allopathic system and Ayurveda belongs to only Ayurvedic doctors. Both sciences are ours and we should not put any one science over the other. It will never ever happen that Ayurvedic medicines cannot benefit allopathic doctors if they take it for their health issue or painkillers of allopathic medicine cannot benefit Ayurvedic doctors for their personal need or to their patients. If medicines are not discriminating and considering all human beings as same, we should think once again before having such prejudice in our minds. Both sciences should work coherent to human health and serve humanity. I am not against modern science, my point is if any science is hurting or working against human health than that science must be avoided where it is increasing human sufferings. Almost every allopathic doctor is familiar with side effects of painkillers, anti-hypertensive medicines, sedative drugs for insomnia, steroids & many more. They knew very well that osteoarthritis cannot be healed with glucosamine, diacerein or NSAID tablets; in fact these medicines will cause renal & hepatic (liver) disorders. Still they are not admitting, this is my point of concern here.

Ordinary people are learning extra ordinary science:

This is the biggest problem with Ayurveda. Ayurveda is highly scientific and advanced system of healthcare. There is no such disease which is not described in original Ayurvedic text, along with its detailed diagnostic criteria and treatment. But the biggest problem is with the way this text is written, if we look only 100 years back we can witness the evolutionary changes in the language of human beings. But as far as Ayurveda is concerned, it is more than five thousand years ancient science. The difference in their language is the biggest issue. Everybody is making translations according to their own mental level. This is the reason why this science is being spoiled by most of the Ayurvedic physicians. Not only this, but most of the teachers who are teaching this science in Ayurvedic institutions have no clue what kind of science is this. This is the reason some group of stupid

Ayurvedic doctors are begging to the government for allowing them to practice basic allopathic medicine. They can neither become a specialist in allopathic system nor are they demanding for that. They just wanted to become a general practitioner & this is the major issue of worry. Our Ayurvedic institutions are failing to teach Ayurveda in such a worst manner that their students are feeling proud to practice like a non-qualified quack. This is like a boy possessing a car is crying to get permitted to drive another vehicle which doesn't belongs to him and not even better from his own car in any sense. On one hand, Ayurvedic doctors are expecting respect from the society and on the other hand, they are shouting to practice in another system. We really need some significant personalities in this field who can teach Ayurveda in a practical way.

Let me bring an example before you, to show how Ayurveda is fundamentally being misunderstood. Brain needs mainly two nutrients to work efficiently. First one is ketones (which are a byproduct of fat) & second one is glucose. Ketones are required in relatively high dose and glucose is important but not required in a huge quantity. Increased level of stress hormone, which is produced from adrenal glands, damages brain and its function, so the nut shell story is high fat, sufficient glucose & minimum stress hormone are basic three ingredients to keep brain healthy and heal various kind of mental disorder. This concept belongs to latest discoveries in our modern science. Before 2010, we were not having this kind of approach towards mental disorders. This science is so new to the medical world that most of doctors are still practicing in their old style of medicating mental disorders. Instead of giving high fat for ketones, some herbs or anti-oxidants to reduce stress level & advising low glucose producing diet, they are still using SSRI, Valproic acid, Eption and other such drugs for their patients which is very harmful. Now, what if I say that this concept which is very latest discovery of medical science was explained in Ayurveda's text book which was written almost 5000 years ago? Ayurveda advises to use some kind of medicated ghee, herbs of "Medhaya" category like licorice root powder, to treat mental disorders. In modern science, also licorice roots & Ashwagandha are now identified as adaptogenic herbs which reduce stress hormone level by supporting adrenal glands. Medicated ghee will produce highly potent ketone bodies in blood & fasting which is called "Langhana" in Ayurveda, will reduce oxidative stress & excess of glucose level in the body. Along with all this, a procedure called "Shirodhara" is also advised to reduce highly active sympathetic nervous system. But most of the Ayurvedic doctors don't even know the whole science & idea behind treating mental disorders because nobody teaches them the whole story. So, in ignorance they are using only "Shirodhara" as a relaxing therapy. This is how Ayurvedic science is being degraded day by day because of ignorance. Our modern society trusts on either scientific explanation or research. It is an unfortunate truth that Ayurvedic doctors can't explain exactly to their patients how this "Shrodhara" will actually works on them. They will only say we believe in our text which says it is good for mental disorders. Believing on text is a good thing but the textual knowledge they are carrying is also superficial. If your doctor is not exactly sure that what is the exact cause of illness than his treatment will always be either superficial or incomplete. Definitely, this will delivers some relief to the patient but without addressing the exact cause it could not be cured permanently.

Let me clear you:

~Any kind of vacuum suction pumps; doesn't belongs to Ayurveda.

~Getting an oil massage in a solo cabin with gentle music in the background; doesn't belongs to Ayurveda.

~Marama Chikitsa is now presented as acupressure, pricking some points with needle for pain relief maybe helpful but that is not Marama Chakitsa. Marama Chakitsa is not even close to acupressure.

~Healing with some kind of invisible radiations or chanting is not Ayurveda either.

~Skipping meal and eating only fruits maybe helpful; doesn't belongs to Ayurveda.

Similarly, there are many treatments that are being referred by some professionals as authentic Ayurveda; maybe something else, but not always Ancient Authentic Ayurveda.

Belief system is degrading Ayurveda:

Believe & trust sounds like same words but it has very big difference. Ayurveda is authentic science and we trust each and every word to be true. This trust should not be spoiled with our own belief system. Everyone who is identified as an Ayurvedic doctor must represent Ayurveda in its original form. Nobody has right to impose his own thought into it & then try to present it as an Ayurvedic concept, because if we start changing the text as per our own belief; we are dis-respecting such a divine science. I am not saying that you must obey whatever is written over there, I am just saying, if you want to change any concept because of your culture, nation or religious belief. Don't forget to present it as your own thinking rather than putting the label of Ayurveda over it.

For example- Ayurveda promotes and supports strongly use of non-vegetarian diet. In the whole text, you can see that Ayurveda advises the use of "Mans Rasa" which is something what we can relate with non-veg. soup or bone broth at many places to treat various diseases. Ayurveda also states that only pasture raised mutton or chicken should be consume; in original text this is called "Jangal Pardesh Mans". Ayurveda has described in detail various wonderful health benefits which include neurogenic disorders, retarded health status after long disease, tuberculosis, vigor, vitality & longevity. But many doctors can be witnessed polluting this concept on the name of Ayurveda just to support their personal belief. If their belief is not allowing them to do so, then they are free to be vegetarian (which is an admirable thing) but they should not say that they trust Ayurveda word by word. They should better say, we disagree Ayurvedic concepts at some places otherwise we are supporter of Ayurvedic concepts. But doing some kind of superstition on the name of Ayurveda is an offence before the creator of this Holy Scripture. Being an Ayurvedic physicians, we all know that this scripture was introduced on this earth by "Lord Dhanvantri" not only this, when this whole incident was happening, we call it "Churning of the ocean" all the three super forces of this whole universe were also present at that time. These three super forces are BHRAMA, VISHNU and MASHESH called creator, administrator & destroyer respectively. So, please rethink what you are saying here; that all of them made a mistake many times in this whole text by advising non-vegetarian diet again & again for different benefits and as a medicine in different disorders. Not only this, let me surprise you that Ayurveda has mentioned proper way & atmosphere to consume alcohol. In original text, word "Sura-paan" is used for drinking. Its dose, time, company describing who can join you, what kind of clothes you should wear while drinking, what kind of music should be played in background almost everything is described in very detail regarding consuming alcohol. Adverse effect will only occur if you dis-obey the rules. Now personally, I am not a drinker but I always explain to those who used to drink that you must follow Ayurvedic rules as mentioned in original text. We are not intelligent or we don't have that understanding level towards body & health as compare to the creator of Ayurveda. While practicing Ayurveda; personal beliefs should be kept aside because it will alter the knowledge concealed in Ayurvedic text.

Not only this, belief system has altered the perception regarding original Ayurvedic text in many ways. Let's take another example of fruits. Most of the doctors and health consultants are recommending fruits as a power house of vitamins, and minerals. Modern science is also supporting this idea and our Ayurvedic doctors are also in this flow. In fact, consuming greens & fruits is believed as an Ayurvedic way of life. Those Ayurvedic doctors who says Ayurveda supports fruits & believe fruits as a healthy habit needs to read Ayurvedic text again. You will be surprised to know that Ayurveda didn't talk much about fruits; Ayurveda only emphasis on vegetables, pulses, ghee, non-veg, certain types of rice (not white & polished rice which we are consuming today). After 2015, many studies has revealed and finally making such health statements which are in a parallel line with ancient Ayurvedic concepts. The knowledge available in Ayurvedic text is so advanced that modern science after spending million dollars on research is proving that right. Now, researchers are explaining that excess of sugar in fruits is actually not healthy. Modern researches never said that fruits are dangerous in little amount also same as with Ayurveda.

Ayurveda also never explained fruits as unhealthy or harmful. Only the perception which says that fruits are very healthy and fruit juices should be consumed regularly is not a good idea. Now let's look at vegetables and fruits in detail. Fruits are majorly water & sugar. It has very little amount of vitamins and minerals in diluted form.

Same minerals and vitamins could be acquired through vegetables & in highly concentrated and heavy amount. Vegetables are also very low in glucose which doesn't spike the insulin response in the body after consuming it. Not only this; Ghee, whole rice (not polished), pulses, non-veg. are also believed & proved healthy as per latest studies. All this is exactly the same as advised in ancient Ayurvedic text. This is the authenticity and trust-ability of Ayurvedic text which should not be altered or ignored.

There are many other things which are misidentified in Ayurveda; one of them is what this whole world knows as "Kerala Panchkarma". I admit that southern part of India has least effect of modernization & modern medicine. They are promoting and practicing Ayurveda in an appreciable manner. But many Ayurvedic doctors in rest of India are trying to mimic them, which is very shameful act. Not only this, they are even trying to pronounce & name medicines and other procedures as it is being spoken in southern states of India. Such activities are a proof that what kind of ordinary minded person are being passed out every year from Ayurvedic medical colleges. When a native doctor of southern states practices Ayurveda in their local style, it is really admirable because 5000 years old language creates a communication gap in today's world. So, it is really their intelligence to practice Ayurveda which sounds native to that particular region. On the other hand, look at those mentally handicapped doctors whose perception is so narrow towards Ayurveda that they are using a mixture of Sanskrit language and southern language in northern part of India which really sounds dumb to me because in this northern part language and culture is totally different. It is not only Kerala Panchkarma it's actually "Ayurvedic Panchkarma". Ayurveda is native to old undivided Punjab which includes today's Punjab along with bigger section of Haryana & Himachal state of northern India. In Ayurvedic text, it is clearly written that Ayurveda is originated in "Panch-nad Pardesh" which means a land of five rivers which is ancient Punjab region of India. Himalayan hills are described as "Aushad Garbha" means creator of Herbal Medicines. But in these areas some doctors are trying to complicate things by altering the names of medicines, Ayurvedic Medical procedures and even the names of their clinics, also sounds like native to southern parts. Southern states are more successful in Ayurvedic practice because they have intelligently decoded Sanskrit language which sounds like their local language and it connects local people to that pathy very easily. No comments for those who are trying to practice Kerala Panchkarma in northern India.

****

Chapter – 8
Fat: Fantastic or Fatal

Fats were integral part of human life since ages. Every culture, every civilization has fat as an important ingredient in their dietary habits in different form. Some civilizations were dependent upon animal fat as their main fat source, while others were dependent on coconut oil or other kind of oils for their healthier living. In India ghee "Clarified Butter" was graded as a super food or best source of fat for healthy living. It was not only included in diet but also been a part of various festivals, celebrations and even in spiritual practices. This represents the understanding of ancient Indian people regarding the importance of fat and its tremendous benefits to health. We managed to survive and lead a healthy life for many thousand years with ghee as an ingredient in almost everything. Nobody was even familiar with cardiovascular disorders, high blood pressure, cholesterol, or any other diseases. Not only India this kind of health status were almost everywhere. There was no fear in the society regarding fat consumption & they were spending a many folds better life as compared to our today's world. Fat causes heart disease; this fear has started from a bogus research conducted by an American physiologist named 'Ancel Keys' (this study is discussed in detail in last chapter of this book). This study was not fact based but actually it's all a decorated research just to prove what they believe. This study was initially rejected by most of the physicians at that time, but unfortunately this report somehow became popular & was published by "Time" magazine in 13 January 1961. After this, low fat era started, we were forced to believe that refined oils are heart healthy, saturated fats are dangerous. Coconut oil is like poison to heart. This is the reason that we have witnessed such a dark age in healthcare because of this misinformation. After 1961, we had increased heart diseases drastically with our so called heart healthy refined oils. Low fat diet has made us obese, mental health has also fallen down very significantly as Alzheimer, behavior disorders, mania & other mental disorders raised worldwide with this low fat diet.

But now, research confirms that we were wrong to understand cholesterols. USA was publishing lots of bad nutritional advises over the years & our so called educated doctors along with other health advisors were also believing USA studies. If they use bit of common sense, they must have questioned themselves that how they can trust on a country who is consuming most unhealthy diet called "Standard American Diet". Believing such a country which is having highest rate of heart diseases, Neurological disorders like Alzheimer, maximum number of USA population is suffering from Diabetes and obesity, should never have been ringed in their minds that can we blindly trust studies from such country who is struggling with life style disorders so badly.

No evidence still exists to prove that having high level of cholesterol causes heart diseases. Recently published study in "Expert review of clinical pharmacology" shows that most of the heart attack patients were shown to have lower than normal cholesterol levels. Doctors continue to promote this lie because this is all what they know. They don't know the whole story, they are just prescribing some pills because they have drug to lower cholesterol. Doctors are paid to prescribe pills, and not to teach how to become healthier. But, I really don't consider doctors as culprits. They are innocent; they really don't know how fats & other nutrients work in the body. Most of doctors who are recommending zero fat diet to our society are overweight and blotted. Their idea of zero fat diet has affected their patients and even to themselves very badly.

Let's talk about some myths & fact related to fats.

Fat will make us obese & worsens diabetes?

This is the first thought anyone will have in his head regarding fat. Fats are believed to make us fat because our society is used to see this in every advertisement. Let's keep logics away for a while and use your common sense. Elephants and buffaloes are accumulating fats in their body from grass only. Have you seen any elephant or buffalo eating their food with fat like butter or ghee? On the other hand, look at other fat eating animals like lion or tiger. Lions are highly sedentary in nature and still they are not obese, their meal comes from 100 percent saturated animal fat or red meat but you can never see a lion visiting a cardiologist or dietician for his so called faulty eating habit.

Now, let's look at it logically. When we eat anything our body stores that energy in the form of glycogen. This glycogen production is dependent on glucose intake of our body. Anything which contains glucose in a direct or indirect form will be stored as glycogen in body. Direct sources of glucose are refined sugar, various fruits, every sweat dish, soft drinks, beer, alcohol, sugary syrups etc.

Indirect sources contain every carbohydrate and starch source. This list is very long & almost 80 percent of our diet consists of this. Rice, Pasta, Bread, Cookies, Potatoes, every cereals-corn, wheat etc. are source of indirect sugars. That means; when you eat these items your body breaks it down to the level of glucose or monosaccharide and then store it as glycogen. This glycogen is actually the fat of your body. Amount of sugar produced in body is measure on a scale called "Glycemic Index". Anything which is high on glycemic index will produce more glucose in body. If this glucose is not used up by your body, it will be stored as a reserve quota. This fat reservoirs are mainly on shoulders, abdomen and flanks in case of men & in females these reservoirs are abdomen, flanks breasts hips & thighs. Our ancient diet was very low on these glucose producing foods but approximately after 1920 we are continuously increasing our sugar contents in eatables. Ice-Cream, candies, sugar syrups, pastries, cakes, artificially flavored fruit juices, soft drinks are now part of our dietary stuffs.

Even cookies & candies are coated with sugar. This high amount of sugar is impossible to be used by body which results in increasing obesity graph. On one hand, we are increasing obesity with sugar and on the other hand, fats are being blamed for all this. This makes condition even more worsen because fat helps to reduce glycemic index response of any meal. But consuming high sugar & low fat is the deadliest combination for human race. It is not the butter on your bread which is causing obesity but it is the bread itself. Refining our sugar and turning it into white crystals was most unhealthiest invention till date. Because insulin response of this refined sugar is almost double as compare to the natural sugar source & now this refined sugar is everywhere and in very high doses in our today's dietary routine. Tea, coffee, sweat dishes, ice-creams etc. cannot be imagined without this sugar. Obesity is only seen in our modern society which survives on grains, chips, cookies, sweet dishes or desserts etc. Not only this sugars, carbs are a kind of simple food which gets easily digested & absorbed in our system. You will be hungry again within no time. This causes you to crave for more & more food in short intervals of time, contributing to increased glycogen production & its storage. After having a fruit juice, ice-cream or soft drink you will store it quickly and can have some other eatable immediately after this. But this could not happen after having high fat butter loaded meal or any high protein source like chick peas. Because fats and proteins are not only low in glycemic index but they also get digested and absorb very slowly which will postpone your next hunger. On one hand, high fat and high protein diets are not only producing low glucose, but also making us eat less. Fat also generates an impulse of satisfaction which means you will not eat or crave anything after this. On the whole, high fat, high protein and zero or low sugar is the only solution for diabetes & obesity. Every bad thing you have heard regarding fat is a Flat **LIE.**

Bloating & Fat:

When stomach bulges out of the body & feels like tenderness or fullness inside, it is called bloating. Bloating is often confused with fats. When stomach is out you are considered fatty but fat is something else. This condition usually starts from indigestion when it is not treated well it becomes a part of your body. To cure bloating what is commonly advised is mostly useless or even adverse in many cases. Bloating when confused with obesity, creates a fear in mind regarding consuming fats. Most of the patients are advised to take fat free diet like boiled or salad but it usually goes in vain.

Bloating is a disorder related to low bile. Bile is strong digestive enzyme which gets triggered when your food pipe detects fat contents in your food. This bile increases BMR, facilitates peristaltic movement, ensures proper cleaning of intestines and many more functions. When we stop consuming fat in our diet, this bile doesn't come in play & all the functions of bile are affected. Bloating could be treated by taking adequate fat in diet, so that bile could be released from gall bladder and delivers its functions. Consuming fat is helpful to cure your bloated stomach also.

Fat Block Arteries?

This is another myth which is very popular concerning risks of consuming high fat diet. It is believed that taking high fat diet will enter in blood vessels & this fat will block our arteries. It could be a broadly talked myth but science doesn't support it. Nothing could be blocked in our blood vessels because design of our human body is not silly design. Body doesn't allow any harmful thing to enter in blood stream. To understand this, let's dig into the science and fact behind this.

Our cardio-vascular system is very important system of our body each & every organ is connected to the heart through blood vessels. This connection allows blood to flow from heart to every body part. Any kind of interruption in this system can affect body very adversely. Body continuously keeps an eye on every minor & major blood vessel. Any kind of damage to the internal lining of these arteries produces a chemical signal which alerts the body. In order to repair this damaged wall, our body sends LDL (Low Density Lipoprotein) to the injured site for repair purpose. This LDL acts as bandage and stick to the internal lining of that ruptured wall. But, if damage to the internal lining is very high than this repair work goes on layer by layer & a thick layer of fat could be built there. Though, we can see fat there but we must look at the cause also. This kind of block will only be created where there is a damaged blood vessel. Therefore, though fats are seen inside blood vessel but it is not there to create any disease; in fact they are protectors. The artery which is blocked now could have been torn apart if fat doesn't serve its cause. Rather than focusing on fats inside the artery, we must focus on the factors which damages blood vessels. Fats can never block a healthy artery.

Chapter – 9
Invisible Inflammation

Before I start this chapter, I need your special attention because may be Inflammation could not be that what you thinks of it. Neither inflammation is your enemy nor is prolonged inflammation good for you. To make my point more clear, I can say any chronic disease or fatal health condition is actually a type of inflammation. Inflammation is like military activity of your body which is an action against any pathogen, foreign body or damage of tissue. It is basically classified in two sections. First type of inflammation is acute inflammation which affects a particular portion or any joint of the body, whereas chronic inflammation is in the whole body. Acute inflammation is seen clearly as it produces visible sign & draws the attention of both patient & doctors. This usually has direct connection with physical injuring and is not related with diet or lifestyle. In laymen, most of the people knows acute inflammation as an inflammatory condition as it is visible clearly and could be spotted as arthritis, tendonitis, frozen shoulder, tennis elbow, spondylitis etc. This acute inflammation represents tissue damage or other kind of deformity in that particular area. Acute inflammation is a smart response of body to repair that particular area. Body tries to provide extra blood supply around that area to promote healing process. Without inflammation your body can't heal even from a minor damage. Inflammation is not a bad thing which should be suppressed with allopathic medicines. Inflammation is also not a deficiency of some anti-inflammatory drugs or a bad thing which should be fixed by throwing chemical tablets inside the system. Our modern doctors are trained to fix inflammation with NSAID's & Steroids resulting body fails to heal that area resulting that temporary condition converts into a lifelong arthritic condition which keeps on aggravating day by day. This is all, because our modern system works against the healing response of body. Animals suffer more inflammatory incidents as compare to human beings because they have to run all the time for basic things like food, water & shelter. Luckily, those animals don’t visit to any big hospital for such minor injury & within few days they heal up completely. On the other hand, if we medicate those animals with the same allopathic medicines that we humans are taking, they will also develop same joint issues like us.

How Inflammation Works:

This is very important & interesting aspect that how inflammation got triggered and how it heals. When your body detects any kind of pathogen inside the body or tissue damage, inflammatory response is triggered immediately. Body facilitates extra blood supply towards that area to provide that portion with extra W.B.C. required fighting against pathogen or extra-nutrients to repair the damaged tissue because everything is carried inside the blood as blood is the ultimate healer. This increased blood supply in a particular area is witnessed by local swelling, redness around that area & slight temperature raise. In medical world, these three signs are the sign of inflammation. When you have hammer in your hand, everything looks like a nail. Same is the case with modern medicine, as they failed badly to understand inflammation because they see inflammation as a bad thing & trained to suppress inflammation with their chemical hammer called steroids and anti-inflammatory drugs. In their perception, inflammation is not a healing process and they look at inflammation as if body is demanding anti-inflammatory drugs. Modern doctors have no clue that what will happen if they use anti-inflammatory drugs so frequently. The side effects which they know are also very insufficient and false. They were only taught the side-effects of these anti-inflammatory drugs but they have never taught the side-effect, if we stop inflammatory process of body. Let's look at an example to have a bird's eye view over this topic. Assume a patient with minor injury in a joint & he visited his nearby hospital to see his doctor. He complained his doctor about swelling in his joint & difficulty in movement of joint. His ignorant doctor will prescribe him some medicines which will stops this healing, inflammatory response of the body & pain will be gone. After few hours, patient will experience zero pain and start moving that joint frequently. When this unhealed joint is moved & no repair process is going on, this joint pain will strike back within few days & this time the damage will be severe than last time. This unhealed joint will be treated the same way again & again with allopathic medicines. Every time, his doctor has to increase the dose than the previous one & this game will ultimately ends at total damaged joint. So, minor tissue damage of joint will ends ultimately to a joint replacement surgery. This is what this whole model of modern medicine is designed for. This system is not designed to provide health; in fact, it is designed to create more & more customers.

Unhealed Acute Inflammation:

Usually inflammation is a temporary process which is designed to heal a damaged organ quickly. It also restricts the movement of that joint which is an indication of your body not to move that joint while healing is under progress. Body will collect required nutrients from the blood to fix that damaged tissue & within few hours or few days this inflammation will be gone by itself. But if body is deficient of some required nutrients for healing process body will constantly keep trying to heal that portion. But due to lack of required nutrients, this try of body to heal will keep on going and inflammation could not serve its cause, resulting long term unhealed inflamed joint. More adversely, when we take allopathic medicines this nutrient reserve will fall more as nutrients are required again to metabolize chemicals in the form of allopathic medicines. The chances of recovery are lost as nutrients requirement increases many folds.

Such kind of inflammation could be healed easily if we provide proper immobilization and required nutrients to the body. But our society is trained in a way that we should not question our doctors as they have a fake spotless reputation.

Chronic (Invisible) Inflammation:-

Earlier we discussed acute inflammation or the inflammation which is visible in a particular area of body. Acute inflammation is not directly linked with faulty eating habits as usually it is caused by some sort of strain, sprain or injury. On the second hand, chronic inflammation is directly caused by the inflammatory food. I call it invisible inflammation because most of the time this inflammation manifests inside the body as a silent host and keep damaging the system without producing any visible symptoms. Basically, it is caused when free radicals increases in the body due to dietary or pathological reasons. This free radicals influence normal metabolism to a stressful condition or we call it "oxidative stress". Name any chronic disease, the root cause of that disease is inflammation. When arteries or muscles of heart get inflamed, it results in the heart attack. If this inflammation occurs in all the skeletal muscles of the body multiple sclerosis is the final result. Inflammation in kidney causes "Renal failure". Inflammation in brain causes Alzheimer, depression or other psychological disorders, Inflammation of respiratory system causes Asthma, COPD, hay Fever, Bronchitis. Inflammation of bones & joints causes osteoarthritis, Rheumatoid Arthritis or Osteoporosis. Various autoimmune disorders like IBS, crohn's disease, colitis, Lupus & Type I diabetes is a result of chronic inflammation in different organs. Many metabolic disorders could also be related with chronic inflammation like Type-II diabetes, liver disorders etc. So,

Inflammation is the only cause for almost every major disorder. Maybe we have named these diseases differently but inflammation is common in all. When any organ or system starts damaging our anti-oxidants in the body works as repair person and re-fix that organ to keep it in working order. But, if free radicals or damage to the system is more than total quantity of anti-oxidants, our body fails to repair that area which results as prolonged inflammation. In simple words, inflammation is like patch work or repair work in any building, if this repair work is done very easily, the building will be in its working order without any disturbance. Chronic inflammation is when building needs repair and building is temporary close for repair work but workers are not available or if workers are available then workers are not having sufficient material for repair like cement, paint etc. In such condition, the building cannot take charge back to be in working order and this closed building is waiting for repair job to be done. This is the perfect example of inflammation in a simpler way.

Pre-Signs of Chronic Inflammation:

Chronic inflammation shows some typical signs before it get converted into a serious health issue. This could also be called a stage between perfect health and chronic disorder. If these signs are present in anyone this could be considered as clinical sign for chronic disorder. Chronic inflammation is hard to be shown in blood reports because our blood investigations only responds positive once the diseases is developed completely. No lab report can anticipate your health or diseases.

But, if these signs are visible we have an opportunity to avoid bigger disorder. Unfortunately, modern doctors are not trained to heal or recover. They can only wait for a positive lab reports so that they can start their symptomatical treatment, accordingly.

Here I will give you a list of symptoms which could be directly related with inflammatory condition in body:

Puffiness on face, mild swelling around eye orbit, hair fall, puffiness in legs, weak digestion, dull face, anxiety, minor headache, weakness & muscular fatigue, irritability, increased urine, disturbed bowl habit either constipation or IBS like symptoms. These are some general signs for inflammatory condition. Some typical symptoms of inflammation which I use in clinical practice is 1) Redness & puffiness in nasal septum without any external factor. 2) Sometimes face shows dis-symmetry between left & right side.

If such symptoms occur, undoubtedly it is a severe inflammatory condition. Though I don't rely blindly on blood reports, still if anyone is not having expertise over clinical signs and language of body than this inflammation could be seen as C-reactive proteins in blood reports. This C-reactive protein or CRP is an inflammatory marker in our body, higher the inflammation in the body; higher the levels of CRP will be found in body. Most of the doctors only know it as a test for arthritis but actually it is an inflammatory marker and it responds to any kind of inflammation in the body. Ideally, it should be less than 2 (two) and if it goes up over 5 (five), risk is there. CRP above 10 is an indicator of high risk from chronic disease.

Inflammatory Foods:

Chronic Inflammation is caused mainly by inflammatory foods. In today's world, it's hard to find unprocessed, non-chemical added, GMO free and organic food. Most of our food creates an inflammatory response that's why majority of our population is under chronic inflammatory condition or diseases related with inflammation. The list of inflammatory food is very long but I will name most common and highly inflammatory foods which must be avoided.

1) Refined - hydrogenated cooking oil.
2) Wheat & other grains containing gluten.
3) Rest over, refrigerated or preserved food.
4) Posturized & homogenized milk.
5) Refined sugar & artificial sweetener.
6) Soft drinks & beer.
7) Bread, Pasta & cheese.
8) Fried and micro-wave heated food stuffs.
9) Canned, packed & preservative added foods.
10) Night Shade vegetables which includes tomatoes, potatoes, eggplant, cyne-pepper, capsicum etc.

Health Mantra's we should learn from animals:

Though we human beings tap our back for drastic development in healthcare sciences but in reality this healthcare system is ruining our health & wealth. Look at ourselves, we visit hospital with money in both hands & come back with bundle of reports in one hand & a bag full of medicines in other hand. Forget bigger health disorders; let's talk about minor health problems and approach of allopathic medicines over it. They are not capable of treating simple gastritis problem permanently, only they can give you a handful of medicines to be taken daily for the rest of your life. And you have no other option except following the same sick trend. Not even single allopathic doctor can answer you exactly that how it is possible, with increasing age when whole body is working slow, our stomach starts producing more HCL acid. Isn't it against the flow of nature, how is it even possible that with age every organ is getting weakens and stomach start producing excess acid surprisingly. They will firstly try to avoid your question. When you insist them for answer, they will try only to blame you for this simple hyperacidity problem. They can't reply you logically that why someone having severe problem of gastritis, has to take some medicines for hyperacidity regularly. Even if he improves his diet as per doctor's advice completely, acidity will still persist. Doctors are charging consultation fees even without consulting and answering their patients. When such advanced system of healthcare is crashing so badly, than we must get inspiration for healthy life from another valid source.

I believe animals have far more respect for nature, health & rules for disease free life. So, I will underline some healthy life style rules which animal kingdom follows and they are far healthier than us. We human beings are such a beautiful, self-healing design of nature which is designed to live on this planet healthy and definitely without consuming colorful allopathic medicines daily. Let's have a look on animals and their health secrets.

Animals never eat after sunset:

Biggest cause of disease is we have forgotten eating time. Sunset is the best time for having last food of the day. Our body also indicates us by striking hunger in the evening. Body tells you that this is the time to eat but we over look that urge and engulf some junky crap at this time and shifts our dinner late night. This culture is biggest reason for our maximum illnesses. Having meal after sunset causes inflammation in body, we look aged earlier, and we disturb hormone alignment of our body by disturbing biological clock.

Early to sleep and early to Rise:

Except owl and bats, most of the animals have strict rule regarding sleeping and waking up. We must know human body is just a speck of this universe. In order to keep this system of body working accurately, we must live in a harmony with this universe. Nights are meant to sleep and with first ray of sun, we must get up. From last few decades, we are cheating this law for financial, social or other reasons. Some people only cheat this law for being so called Modern. But modernization is always about advancement not retrogressiveness. Anything which benefits you and comforts you should be called modern and vice-versa. But we are tagging inferior eating, damaging lifestyle and flawful things as modern. Anything which is hurting human body and life is called modern these days.

Modern medicine, modern culture, modern lifestyle, modern food & many more modern things are actually not modern.

Animals don't eat in sickness:

This is another golden rule which animal follows but we are unaware of it. When we are sick or we suffer from fever, best remedy is to stop eating anything. Your body also wants you not to eat during sickness. When we stop eating, our body can use its all energy for recovery process but when we keep eating small meals or anything like fruits or juice, our body has to divide its energy in healing and digestion process at the same time; which increases the recovery time. Digestion, absorption is very big and significant process for our body. We can see only digestion but we don’t even know thousands of biochemical pathways which get activated behind the scene, when we eat anything. Water fast is the best way to fight with fever or another minor health issues.

Re-eating, over-eating and snacking:

We human beings are social animals & this socialism is above everything, even above from our health. It is often seen that after having a full meal, we can accept any kind of sweet dish, cookies or any other eatable. But this is not the case with animals. Once they are done with eating, it means they are done. You can't insist your dog for another bite of food after he eats his food with satisfaction. This is very important point because throwing food after food makes your food like a poison. Food is only going to benefit you, if, it is well digested and well absorbed. Undigested food produces poisonous chemicals which is dangerous in many ways to our body.

Last but not the least; Animals are not dependent on allopathic chemical based medicine to fix or to suppress their health issues.

We must have this basic sense that anything which is not the constituent of our body or any unnatural substance is harmful for our system. Allopathic medicines are strong chemical base medicine and they are not constituent of our system. These medicines increase our diseases day by day by suppressing only symptoms. These chemicals not only shortens your life but also gifts you some latest trending diseases with lots of side-effects or in more simpler way it could be said that we buy diseases and side-effects at very expensive rates. When we visit any hospital for general disease, everyone is getting economic benefit from your pocket and you carry back some fancy medical terms, poisonous medicines and invitation for new diseases. Allopathic medicine, if really improves your health status then amount of medicine must be decreased with time as patient improves and finally medicines should be discontinued with time but once you start allopathic medicine, the dose and strength has to be increased with time just to keep you going. What does it means, you can imagine this better. This is the reason hospitals are getting bigger & health status is declining day by day.

Science of Rejuvenation:

Since ages, Rejuvenation has been always in limelight. From Vedic era, this topic got a special attention from everyone. Rejuvenation being so vast topic is still basic and natural. Rejuvenation is not a miraculous thing which will happen with some mysterious & miraculous herbs. Most of the pharmaceutical companies & some deceitful Ayurvedic doctors are presenting this topic in a wrong manner. Let me be very clear here, rejuvenation cannot be packed in some kind of fancy capsules, syrups, supplements or tonics. This is basic potential of your body which varies from person to person depending upon dietary, geographical & other factors. A simple wound healing is also rejuvenation of your body. If you get a cut on the body, you never order your body to heal that cut. This is body's own ability to heal that cut by its own. All the bandages, septic solutions or other tablets are just to avoid pathogen attack on that exposed area. All this stuff works only on securing that cut from pathogen attack. They have nothing to do with healing of that cut. Healing is body's own ability.

When we talk about anti-aging & other related aspects of rejuvenation we must know that this is also body's own ability. Breakdown of body is a natural phenomenon, mountains, forests, rocks everything on this planet ages with time. Even our whole planet earth is also continuously changing & aging with time. Only we can do is to slowdown this ageing process or speed-up recovery. Aging and rejuvenations is dependent on the ratio of breakdown & recovery or we can say free radicals & anti-oxidants ratio. Increasing free radicals in diet will definitely give a rejuvinatory effect to the body.

But, if we can manage to reduce damage of the body or free radical load & simultaneously increasing anti-oxidant level within the body; the rejuvenation could be shoot very high. Everything in your body is designed to heal itself then why in osteoarthritis case, we assume that meniscus of the joint could not be healed. We are so brain washed by modern, medical system that we look at everything as per the range of allopathic medicinal system. This is true that allopathic medicines cannot heal joint in arthritis but this doesn't means that your body is not designed to heal. We have two different departments in rejuvenations; first one is having proper nutrients available within the body to rebuild that joint and second is body's hormonal alignment required for healing. Every organ takes particular time to regenerate by itself, the only condition is body must have required raw material (nutrients) for healing and regeneration. If favorable condition is given; bones & joints can replace itself completely within one year. Which means after one year you will have a new bone in your body as old bone will be replaced with new bone cells completely. Now the question is, in osteoarthritis why bone is being replaced with damaged joint again? This is because your doctor is treating osteoarthritis with standard calcium tablets, NSAID's, steroids & maybe with a blood thinner; if you complaints your doctor for high blood pressure. If you are on such medicines, forget rejuvenation, you are damaging your system very quickly now because your joint doesn't need this chemical crap to rebuilt itself. This is like your car mechanic needs engine oil & some necessary wiring to repair your car but you are offering him milk, phenyl, alcohol, cookies & all such non-relevant stuff. Whose fault is this?

Similarly liver is the fastest healing organ of our body but allopathic doctors keeps medicating liver disorders for years. They don't have idea how this body works. What your body requires in a healthy state and which nutrients are required to heal a particular system of the body. That's why I say, "God Bless Modern Medicine".

Clinical aspects of rejuvenation:

Anything which is described as inflammatory food must be avoided. Lifestyle habits must be disciplined to promote better functioning of the body. Every food which causes inflammation produces free radicles in the body and freezes rejuvenation must be excluded from diet. Diet must be saturated with anti-oxidants and all the required essential 90 nutrients to the body in proper proportion.

This rule of rejuvenation is applied to all the systems of the body; give that system required nutrients in the form of herbal medicines & keeps nourishing body regularly for a certain time, you can heal every disorder.

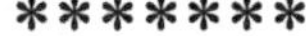

Chapter – 10
Allopathic Reductionism V/s wholistic Approach

Before I proceed further in this topic, let me define two basic fundamental concepts or better to call basic principle on which we will be discussing in this chapter.

What we know today as allopathic system was started by 'Hippocrates', who believes what cannot be seen or measured does not exist at all. This is called reductionism. This tells you to increase anything which is low from normal and to decrease that is raised form normal value. Though this theory seems logical at first glance but if we look into this in context with human health this theory works horribly bad. Such theory of reductionism is for simple machines where selected procedures are being performed but not in a complex, highly evolved species like human body, where thousands of bio-chemical reactions are being carried out at same time. Suppressing one system with a chemical tablet can alter many other vital bio-chemical reactions of the body, resulting in serious malfunctioning. Many allopathic doctors I meet doesn't know that their allopathic system is basically designed on principle of reductionism e.g. If there is foul smell in any room of a house, reductionism thinking will say to either spray heavy perfume in that room to suppress that annoying smell or to lock that room & avoid the exposure. I think now reductionism will be understood to my readers.

On the other hand, wholistic system is the law of nature which says everything in universe is connected to each other with an invisible but highly strong thread. Change in any single phenomenon will produce visible changes in every other system also. 'Wholistic' term comes from word 'whole' which means all in one. Similarly, inside our body uncountable reactions are taking place which we cannot even discover. This is the wisdom of that almighty creator. Reductionism theory does not believe in soul, rebirth or any such stuff but they can never explain everything stop working once a person is dead, what was that energy by which all those reactions were being driven. Nothing goes away from the body after death according to reductionism then why we cannot cheat death by restarting every function of the body.

I like this word "quack":

Before I go in details about this word "quack", let's uncover when this was started. In 1901, a person named "Simon Flexner" who was director of 'Rockefeller Institute for medical research'. This was the year, when this Institute was founded. After three years in 1904, American Medical Association created a council for medical education; regarding this, huge money was required. Henry Pritchett (President of Carnegie foundation) take over this whole council of medical education (C.M.E.) then this man (Henry) sent Abraham Flexner for a survey in the country regarding medical colleges. This Abraham Flexner was brother of Simon Flexner (director of Rockefeller Institute for Medical Research). Now I want you to make a link here that what were the connection before this whole story of allopathic takeover of medicine. Because when this Flexner report was submitted in 1910 they used this report as a base to call everyone a "quack" except allopathic doctors. Before 1901 there were different types of medical schools doing fantastic work like homeopathy, naturopathy & chiropractic. But in between 1901 & 1910, money played an important role to take over every established & authentic system of medicine. Not only this, they even called them all “a quack” & start blowing there on trumpet till date. My apologies for this story which might make you bored but truth also deserved to be uncovered.

1) Allopathic doctors blocks digestion with proton pump Inhibitors & quacks improve digestion.
2) Allopathic doctors find suitable tablet to suppress high blood pressure & quacks find reason for high blood pressure.
3) Allopathic doctors try to treat human body with synthetic chemicals which is even poisonous for plants whereas quacks uses only natural substances for medicating.
4) Allopathic doctors believe that every system works independently but quacks knows body as a single unit.
5) Allopathic doctors study effect of medicines on a particular system, quacks studies nutrition before studying natural medicines.

6) Allopathic doctors changes medicine with symptoms quacks find reason for that symptom and changes lifestyle to avoid unnecessary medicines.
7) Allopathic doctors start, anti-hypertensive medicine which finally ends at either various system damage or cardiac bypass surgery. Whereas quacks are not so skilled to perform bypass surgery, so they prefer to cure the disease permanently and that hypertension, anti-cholesterol medicines, blood thinness could be avoided because they can damage heart.
8) Allopathic doctor looks at cholesterols as a terrorist which can attack heart. So they immediately start attacking heart and cholesterols both at the same time with their chemical weapons like statins, blood thinners, ACE-Inhibitors etc. On the other hand, quacks looks at cholesterol as a raw material which body is producing itself for various needs like production of progesterone & testosterone, cortisol, repair of different tissues of body like skin or brain cells.
9) Allopathic doctor believes that diluting blood with a chemical is very good idea where as quack looks blood as a river of life which nourishes whole body by its nourishing and healing property.
10) Allopathic doctors are smart enough to kill the mosquitoes (pathogens) produced over the garbage inside the body but dumb quacks clean the garbage permanently.

I had eaten an alternative food today:

Allopathic hypocrisy says only we are doctors and only we deals in authentic medicine, rest of all the pathies are alternate. Now, this is strange to me; without allopathy human generations lived healthy and managed to survive generations after generation. But only from last hundred years after the allopathic take over, everyone knows where our health status is going. With due respect to allopathic system I just want to say every system is a healthcare system. No matters if it is naturopathic system, Chinese herbs, Ayurvedic system of medicine, chiropractic or homeopathy. They all are sciences and have their stronger and weaker sides. I always thank allopathy for emergency care, trauma care, advanced surgeries & anti-biotic like penicillin, but we must admit allopathic works horribly wrong while treating life style disorders, general health ailments and many more.

We must have this common sense in our minds that every food of different countries or religion is a food. Every food serves its cause very well and no-one can deny its importance. But imagine a guy who is eating chemical tablets for everything. He claims that his chemical food is evolved after many researches and trials on rats. He is eating a tablet for each nutrient like carbohydrate, protein, fats, minerals & he is still doing well with his life. No-one has problem with this but, suddenly this guy start shouting that he is eating only real food & rest of the people are eating alternative food. This is the same story with medicine also, we never criticize if you are promoting your chemical base medicine but should we keep silence if you are calling yourself as real doctors and rest of all as "a quack", only your medicine is verified medicine & rest of all are practicing alternative medicine. Sorry! I refuse to acknowledge your perception.

Only reason that allopathic doctors are on front foot today:

We must understand every system is driven and influenced by money. No-one cares how effective, beneficial or healthy food is it, if it cannot benefit economically, no-one will promote it and it is a fact. We all know the benefits of lime water but advertisement will sell you toxic soft drinks with little flavor of lemon & a big picture of lemon on the label. No-one will advise you to take freshly made lemon water at home in their advertisements. Big companies are also selling & advertising hypothetical health benefits of red colored syrup with chemical flavor of pomegranate. They will never tell you that fresh pomegranate fruit from local farmer's market is healthy for you. No-one can advertise & promote original thing because it costs more & producer cannot give economic shares to these advertisements whereas mixing chemical in a bottle with added artificial sugar is cheaper than anything, so this could generate profit. Same is the case with allopathic medicines because these medicines are also chemical base. It costs nothing to manufacturer but it is sold at very higher prices. This is the reason that allopathic industry is capable enough to be always in lime light. Televisions are showing them, corporate hospitals are hiring them, insurance companies are only covering bills of allopathic medicines, newspapers are publishing them & people are forced to believe that only allopathy is the real pathy which cares about life. But, from last 15-20 years the result of this lie is making big noise. In last 15-20 years, health statistics is broken like hell, we are facing explode of lifestyle disorders like diabetes, obesity, hypertension, auto-immune disorders & many more. Because the pathy everyone trusted has zero knowledge about lifestyle & nutrition. This pathy is only good at nomenclature as it names simple health disorders in very complex medical terms that the people feels that they know something significant. If a person visit a doctor with pain in foot and he asks doctor for diagnosis. Medical doctor may call it "Metatarsalgia" & the patient will trust the academics of that doctor. But now, if we dig into this term this isn't diagnose, it is just paraphrasing in medical terminology. Literally his doctor is saying pain in foot because metatarsalgia is made from two words metatarsals & algia. Meta-tarsal is a bone of foot & algia stands for pain. Congratulations! you have the diagnosis now, you must start regular therapy of pain-killers, steroids etc.

If all the pathies given equal opportunities, same government support, same insurance benefits then within five years, not only these medical doctors will be out of business but health statics will thanks the society for this necessary change. This change will confine all allopathic doctors only up to surgery, trauma care & chronic infections in which they are good. At last, let me speak again that I am not against allopathic system because it has its stronger sides also. I am only against the culture which is promoting false information which is not only against human health but also against science, bio-chemistry and physiology of the body.

If you can't create a human life then you have no right to hurt it with you chemical medicines only for economic reasons and suppressing symptoms.

The research you trusted could be biased; the facts you know could be a Myth:

Since this modern science is always believed to be evolved from many researches and data study. So everyone trusts this pathy blindly without hesitation. But this is also not true every time. I am only underlining the point that even if the information is coming after long research still it could be flawful.

The research you trust could be biased the fact you know could be a myth.

Since this modern science is always believed to be evolved from many researches and data study. So, everyone trusts this pathy blindly without hesitation. But this is also not true every time. I am not saying that every research is flawful but I am only underlining the point that even if the information is coming after long research still it could be flawful. Let me introduce you here the biggest blunder research of all the time. Since, from last 60 years, we are forced to believe on a lie which says; saturated fats and cholesterol cause heart attack. We have presented a theory which says when we eat fats or saturated fats it gets into our bloodstream and clogs up arteries, resulting in heart attack. They believe that anything which enters inside our stomach gets directly carried up by a blood vessel which is very idiotic idea. Blood composition is dependent on totally different science and bio-chemical needs of body. Let's assume this theory is true for a while that taking fat in diet enters our blood then definitely one day apple, spinach and other food stuffs could also be found in our bloodstream. This lie of taking saturated fat causes heart attacks is started by an American physiologist "Ancel Benjamin keys" and "TIME Magazine" cho0osed to devote his cover page to this researcher. Since then, all the doctors till date is following that notion in their heads, that fats are dangerous for health. Though there were many flaws with the method of the research process but still it gained publicity and this lie is so big today. This fear from fat is not easy to erase because we are living with this lie from last 60 years. In 2014, "American Heart Association" also cleared that there is no valid evidence which can prove that fat can cause heart disease but still doctors are stuck in that old fat fear tradition. Not only had this, "Time Magazine" itself placed a "Butter slice" on its cover magazine in 2014 to explain the health benefits of taking fat. But, I believe our conventional doctors are like old "Pentium Processor' Computers" which are unable to refresh by its own and got hanged over the old concepts. Logically speaking, after 2014 almost all popular sources refused to label fats for any health disorder but hardly anyone is talking about it even today. There were many methodological flaws in the research work of "Ancel keys" but I'll mention few of them.

Initially, this research was conducted in 22 different countries, but after studying all 22 countries only 7 countries were considered in the final submission report because rest of the countries was not proving his perception right. He cheated his own report very cleverly, just to prove his personal belief. Rest of the 15 countries was taking high fats diets and was healthy. Germany, France and some other European countries were not included in the final submission report of his research.

This research was actually based on co-relation and not causation. Research is only meant to be a controlled research, which means research can clearly prove that one particular thing is causing another and if we continues first thing then second will vanishes away by its own. But, this was not happening with "Ancel's" research. He just looked at co-relations simply & framed a hypothetical diagnosis, which could hardly be true. Let me explain this for making my point more transparent. Looking at only co-relation can went horribly wrong because it does not prove first thing causing other, what these kind of research can prove is merely a coincidence for example: in a particular year by looking at a line graph, it could be co-related that sales of four-wheeler vehicles and divorce rate increases in a parallel pattern. But we all know, sales of four wheeler vehicles cannot influence divorce rate in a country, this is simply a case of co-incidence. This is just an example that how co-relating can drastically went wrong.

"Ancel keys" report was not even done in a favourable environment. The candidates who were chosen for this research work was not only taking fats but also consuming the refined, preserved, trans-fat added and anti-inflammatory, un-healthy food at the same time. How could they prove that the deaths were only related with unsaturated fats and not because of other faulty eating habits?

Myth and facts:

Myth: Saturated fats like red meat, coconut oil, MCT oil, butter etc. are dangerous to health.

Fact: Saturated fats are actually important for our body. Skin, GIT, brain cells, vital organs are actually made up from saturated fats. All these organs need saturated fats for its repair and maintenance. Saturated fats are considered toxic because of 'Ancel keys' biased research work only. Other than that, no-one has any valid proof to recognize saturated fats as culprits.

Another reason for consuming saturated fats is your body's fundamental unit 'cell'. We all are just a bunch of cells in a particular arrangement; our cell membrane is also made up of phospholipid bilayer with some proteins embedded in it. Even this cell membrane is a phospholipid, which is a saturated fat structure, what else reason you could have to include saturated fats in diet? If our very basic structure of body is made from saturated fats then how could it be claimed that these types of fats are harmful for us? Think over it again with a logic and scientific point of view.

Myth: Fruits are very healthy and fruit juices are a super drink loaded with health.
Fact: Though I never considered fruits as a harmful thing but I also believe fruits are over-rated. We have placed fruits at a higher rank than they deserves. Fruits are just a combination of sugar, some vitamins and trace minerals. No doubt, these nutrients are significantly important for human body but the proportion is not really that good. Fruit contains majorly water and sugar in it. Vitamins in fruits and other minerals are only in diluted form. So, fruits are not a good option for those who are in a condition where sugar is not recommended to be consumed, such as: obesity, diabetes, certain mental disorders, metabolic syndrome and many others.

Let's talk about fresh fruit juice; a glass of your fresh fruit juice is majorly water and sugar. You must know, the waste which is thrown out from fruits while preparing juice carries most significant thing called roughage (fibres) with some minerals and vitamins. Which means diluted nutrients of fruits gets even more diluted in your fresh fruit juice glass, as the waste material carries certain amount of nutrients within them. Only exception among fruits is "Indian gooseberry" or what we commonly refer as 'amla'. This is the only fruit which carries all the nutrients in surprisingly high concentrations. That's why, this is the only fruit which is praised a lot in Ayurvedic texts.

Myth: Olive oil is the best form of oil.
Fact: This is another lie, which is being promoted a lot in this modern era. Though olive oil is again not

dangerous oil but many facts are over looked regarding this particular oil.

95 present of olive oil, which is available on supermarket shelves is not actually olive oil either. Olives are very limited on our planet but it is supplied in a huge quantity all over the world now. Olive oil has two main properties which makes it controversial oil in my observation.

This oil has strong tendency to get oxidised, which means after some time this oil will be oxidised by its own. Oxidised oil is a leading cause of oxidative stress and inflammation. This oil is only beneficial, if it is used in very short period after its extraction, which is not possible commercially. No matters, how well you store it or preserved it; oxidation is a natural process and we cannot cheat this process by any method.

This oil has very low smoking point, which is another trouble. Let’s assume, you belong to that area where olives are found and grown. You are capable enough to get this oil in very fresh form before it gets oxidised. Still it is not that all-purpose super oil. It has very limited range of cooking which means it could not be over heated because once it attains its smoking point it will produce toxic carbonic chemicals; which may lead to joint pain, liver disorder, inflammatory condition and even carcinoma (cancer).

In context of cooking; different oils are beneficial for different cooking styles and there is no such super oil which should be called all-purpose supreme oil. In Indian context, mustard oil and ghee is best option. Some traditional south Indian dishes go best with coconut oil. Though in some states of India groundnut oil is also preferred but regular use of this oil is not healthy as it is inflammatory in nature and interferes with liver functions also.

Myth: Hydrogenated oil and vanaspati ghee are safe to use.

Fact- this is most toxic lie you have even heard. Hydrogenated oils are not even for human use but there are many popular brands out in the market selling this toxic grease and promoting it also as heart healthy oil.

This kind of oil was firstly introduced for human use by an American base company with brand named "Crisco". This company is the root source from where all this has started. You might not believe but it is a fact that this company is so good in advertising as it convinced the people to believe, what they are selling is healthy. This company is still in business today.

Any kind of refined oil or hydrogenated oil is not good for your body or your heart either. This kind of toxic oils is only good for the pocket of your cardiologist.

Anyhow, I hope my points against that research are sufficient to break your belief system on research regarding fat fear. At last I just want to say that treating spinal disorders with Lumbo-sacral belts and painkiller or knee pain with a knee cuff and steroids is not what we can do. We must look at some authentic treatments, which facilitate healing process of the body and patients can heal permanently. We must stop believing blindly at all our treatment options given by our health science and establish a wolistic approach. The pathy we are trusting is going to meet its dead end soon. In last 100 years our society has seen the lethal effects of this so called old fashioned modern science.

Vaid [signature]

(VAID ATWAL)
10-AUGUST-2019

Enough for this book now, I'll try to come back soon with another topic. Till then, wishing you a healthy and prosperous life; hoping that this book will definitely improve your awareness towards human body.

****

Your feedback is much appreciated
Contact author- ohcc.asr@gmail.com
Follow on
You can also contact author for guest lectures, seminar and conceptual classes on health and disease.
Email id - ohcc.asr@gmail.com
Instagram - Vaid Atwal
Facebook - Vaid Atwal (Facebook Page)
for any kind of have queries and dietary Consultation visit our website
www.vaidatwal.co.in
Special discount package for bulk purchase in libraries and other institutions.
10 copies or above - Only Shipping Will Be Complimentary
50 copies or above- Rs. 70 less on per book cost + shipping extra
100 Copies or Above – Rs. 100 Less On cost + Shipping Extra

CONTACT SANKALP PUBLICATION ONLY FOR BULK SUPPLY.
(9111395888, 9111396888)
(https://sankalppublication.com)

9 789388 660730

Printed by Libri Plureos GmbH in Hamburg,
Germany